LUKE BAILEY REED JR.

VEGETARIAN MEAL PLAN FOR BODYBUILDERS

PLANT-BASED AND HIGH PROTEIN DIET FOR BODYBUILDING ATHLETES, SPORTS ENTHUSIASTS AND BEGINNERS.
LEARN HOW TO BUILD AND INCREASE MUSCLE, BURN FAT AND GET LEAN.

advice. The content within this book has been derived from various sources. Please consult a licensed professional before attempting any techniques outlined in this book.

By reading this document, the reader agrees that under no circumstances is the author responsible for any losses, direct or indirect, which are incurred as a result of the use of information contained within this document, including, but not limited to, — errors, omissions, or inaccuracies.

Contents

CHAPTER 6. HOW MANY MACRO SHOULD I EAT? 115

CHAPTER 7. HOW TO GET THE RIGHT AMOUNT OF PROTEIN AND OTHER BENEFITS FROM A VEGETARIAN DIET? 132

Introduction

Since time immemorial bodybuilders have relied heavily on a high-meat and poultry diet to get the requisite amount of proteins to build muscle mass. However, there is a steady rise in the new wave of bodybuilders who are challenging the traditional norm of getting proteins only from meats and milk and instead are propagating plant-powered food. This new community of bodybuilders believes that with a strict commitment to a plant-based diet and a change in eating habits, one can get enough proteins for bodybuilding. Vegan bodybuilding diet can help in a great way to attain this goal. But before plunging into a full-fledged vegan diet, there are a few tips that can help get started with this regime-

Get enough calories- The most important thing for new vegans is to take enough calories on a regular basis so that the body does not consume incoming protein for fueling body growth. This could lead to a deficit.

Have vegetables and fruits in plenty- It is important to take in a good quantity of fruits and vegetables as they keep up the nutrient content in the body and also provide antioxidants to maintain immunity.

Eat legumes and chickpeas- For vegans looking to build muscle, it is important to consume sufficient quantities of legumes and chickpeas. They are a high source of carbohydrates and make for a tasty snack after a rigorous session of workout.

Switch to quinoa instead of rice- Quinoa is a mixture of brown rice and oatmeal and is higher in the overall content of protein than brown rice. Also, it is a complete protein source, which is essential for muscle building.

Soy protein powder- Include soy protein powder with other natural sources of protein to increase the amount of protein in your body. In fact, it should be a must-have for all bodybuilders.

Avoid processed food- In vegan bodybuilding for beginners' diet, the consumption of processed food is limited. Being vegan does not mean that you can have a free hand at eating any amounts of carbohydrates. Eating healthy is of prime importance with a diet containing nuts, fresh fruits, vegetables, and whole grains.

Have a short but intense workout- As a vegan, you should indulge in short, intense workouts. It will not allow the loss of muscle mass and will let your body rely on vegan protein sources through the workout sessions. It has been seen that long workout sessions often lead to fatigue for vegans in the long run.

Have a varied choice in food you consume- As a vegan, you might find yourselves eating the same food repeatedly. Try to avoid this as it can lead to nutritionally deficiencies and not add to muscle building.

Eat frequent meals- Since you cannot consume as much protein in each meal as a non-vegetarian, you should add more meals to your day so that there is a steady stream of proteins going into the muscles.

Food rich in muscle-building amino acids- Amino acids are the building blocks of tissues and protein in the body. The body requires 21 amino acids to stay alive, and nine are found in food. These are called essential amino acids, and one of them called cinephile is related to muscle-building and it allows protein synthesis in the body through enzyme activation needed for cell growth. Thus, the leucine content in the meal shows the protein content required for muscle building. So eat foods rich in amino acids and especially leucine.

Making these simple lifestyle changes will go a long way in adjusting to the vegan way of life and will allow the proteins to be absorbed well to create as much muscle mass as a non-vegan diet would.

Planning a proper vegan meal

Meal planning is of the utmost importance when undertaking a vegan diet, especially for bodybuilders and athletes.

There are a few things that you need to keep in mind while planning a proper diet-

Calorie Intake- Accurate calorie tracking is the most effective and reliable way to know what is going into the body, how to lose fat, and build muscle. It does not mean starving yourself, but instead, it includes the number of calories you eat and how many you might burn. It is called energy balance.

Work out macros- There are three macronutrients that the body needs- proteins, fats, and carbohydrates. They make up a major part of our calorie intake and the macronutrient split is essential to build a great looking body for bodybuilders. They dictate how the body will grow and repair tissues, and how much muscle you retain during a weight loss program. The optimal vegan macro split should be-

Have a high-protein diet consuming 0.73-1 g per lbs.

Have a low to moderate-fat diet: Get 15-30% calories from fat.

Let the remaining calories be in the form of carbohydrates.

Plan meat timing and portions- Once you have figured out how to split the macronutrients in every meal, it is time to plan your meal timing and also the portion size. Since you are getting all the proteins from plants; it is not feasible to get the requisite amounts in just three main meals of the day. Hence, it is pertinent to add more meals at frequent intervals with substantial amounts of protein in each meal. It will help stoke the metabolic fire and burn more fat. In addition to it, the continuous consumption of protein will help in muscle growth at optimal capacity. The timing of the meal is also important. Late night dinners or might-night snacks are a big no. Stay away from food after sunset or reduce it to minimal.

Plan what foods for each meal- It is important to decide on the kind of proteins you want to have in each meal. So planning each meal with care is significant. Include fresh fruits, nuts, and vegetables on a daily basis. Get the macronutrient split right so that there is a proper percentage of each nutrient for adequate muscle repair and growth.

Chapter 1.
The Vegetarian Diet

The origins of vegetarianism date back to ancient times. But the term «Vegan» was first used in the 40s by Donald

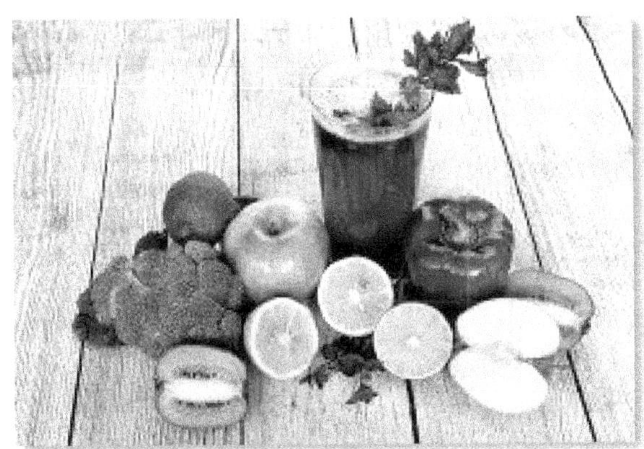

Watson, co-founder of the Vegan Society, to describe a lifestyle doctrine that man should live without exploiting animals.

The following decades saw substantial growth in the industrialization of food production and an increase in the nature of food. We seemed to move from a "garden to plate" life to a 'factory to plate". Food came out of convenient packets, which we threw away after eating the unhealthy contents, resulting in bad health for us and garbage and gasses for the planet.

By the 70s attitudes to health followed a trend toward a more natural lifestyle. Cultures blended many ideas from the East, and food production in western countries came under scrutiny. Along with a movement towards more compassionate living, people started to become critical of meat-eating and the way animals are treated when they are bred for food.

A move towards more natural food production methods for plants and animals started gaining awareness amongst the younger generations, who had to deal with the damage that unhealthy food production was causing to the earth, to plants and animals, and us.

Vegetarianism became a trend a growing trend in the west. But also, we now realize that some cultures have been traditionally vegetarian for thousands of years.

Veganism seems to have evolved from recognizing that even a vegetarian lifestyle still doesn't improve the risk of certain kinds of health issues and that even a vegetarian lifestyle doesn't eliminate the suffering caused to animals when they are used for what they produce. Vegetarianism has become a trend in the West. But also, we now realize that some cultures have been traditionally vegetarian for thousands of years.

The production of eggs still involves the battery farming of chickens. Cows are physically restrained for hours a day, not to mention the diet and medical intervention required to make them produce more milk than they are evolved to produce.

Veganism recognizes that any treatment of animals that raises them for the production of food and products involves some measure of suffering.

We will look at more specific aspects of veganism and a vegan dietary choice in this book.

TYPES OF VEGETARIANISM AND THEIR DIFFERENCES

Veganism and vegetarianism - just words or a way of life?

People often do not understand the difference between vegans and vegetarians.

The reason is that the very concept of vegetarianism is inaccurate and can mean different eating styles. Vegetarianism (from Lat. Vegetarius - vegetable) is a common name for food systems (diets) based on the use of plant products and the exclusion or limitation of the consumption of animal products.

Veganism is a lifestyle based on great moral awareness. The diet itself is only a consequence of the moral and ethical views of veganism. Vegans have special dietary rules, and veganism is often practiced for ethical reasons. Below we look at vegan principles in more detail.

Types of vegetarianism:

- Lacto-ovo-vegetarianism
- Lacto-vegetarianism
- Ovo-vegetarianism
- Veganism
- Raw food diet
- Fruitarianism
- Unusual types of vegetarian diets (Polotarianism, Pescatarism)

LACTO-OVO-VEGETARIANISM

In the modern world, Lacto-ovo-vegetarianism can be called the most common vegetarian diet.

The term Lacto-ovo-vegetarianism itself comes from Latin words: lacto - milk, egg - egg, vegetation - vegetation.

As the name implies, a lacto-ovo-vegetarian diet allows you to use milk and dairy products, eggs and any plant products. Any meat of animals, whether it is meat, poultry, fish or seafood, is excluded from the diet.

As followers of any other vegetarian diet, lacto-ovo-vegetarians are divided into ethical vegetarians who adhere to the vegetarian diet for ethical or religious reasons, and vegetarians who adhere to this diet for the benefit of their health.

If your diet is balanced correctly, then switching to a lacto-ovo-vegetarian diet will be completely painless for you. The fact is that animal products will remain on your daily menu. You can still eat egg and dairy products. Almost all your favorite dishes may well remain on your menu.

A properly planned lacto-ovo-vegetarian diet should include the following products weekly:

6-12 servings of cereal products, cereals, legumes

6-8 servings of dairy products (cheese, milk, cottage cheese, natural yogurt, sour cream, etc.)

4-6 servings of vegetables and vegetable dishes

3-5 servings of fruit

1-2 eggs per day (including eggs that are already found in various foods, such as baked goods).

It is also recommended that you include nuts and dried fruits in your diet. Nuts contain a large amount of protein, phosphorus, zinc, magnesium, iron, calcium, and dried fruits are an excellent source of iron.

LACTO-VEGETARIANISM

The word "Lacto-vegetarianism" consists of two parts. The prefix «lacto-» comes from the Latin word "lactis", which means milk. The second part - vegetarianism - is well known to everyone who is at least to some extent interested in the problem of healthy eating.

It is also the most popular course among vegetarians.

Lacto-vegetarianism is a vegetarian diet that, in addition to vegetable products, allows you to consume milk and dairy products, whether it is cheese, cottage cheese, butter, etc. But lacto-vegetarians may not eat all kinds of cheeses. Cheeses that contain an enzyme of animal origin, such as abomasum, are excluded from the diet.

Lacto-vegetarians exclude from their diet all products of animal origin, including eggs, only dairy products are allowed. Dairy products in this form of nutrition are the main source of protein.

To a large extent, lacto-vegetarianism is ethical vegetarianism. People on this diet believe that products of animal origin can be used, but only if they are obtained by non-violent means.

Due to the presence of milk and dairy products in this diet, the content of such important substances as, for example, calcium, vitamin D and vitamin B12, will be sufficient, and you will not need to consume large amounts of nutritional supplements.

Also, thanks to dairy products, you can be sure that your body receives all the necessary amino acids.

OVO-VEGETARIANISM

Ovo-vegetarianism is a type of vegetarianism excluding all animal products except eggs.

Like lacto-vegetarians, ovo-vegetarians are convinced of the need to eat animal protein and, in particular, an egg.

But there is one important point - you can eat only unfertilized eggs. If the eggs are fertilized, then a new life has already begun in it, which cannot be killed.

VEGANISM

People who are, or have been vegetarian for a long time, think switching to Veganism is easy. After all, you have not eaten meat or animal products for ages. Then you reach for the honey to sweeten your tea and realize that the vegan life means no honey or milk in that steaming mug of tea.

So honey is a "No", but what about silk from silkworms or makeup using animal by-products?

Veganism is a lifestyle based on great moral mindfulness. The diet itself is only a consequence of the moral and ethical views of veganism.

Veganism as a diet has a very large ethical component. This is the case when people are primarily guided by humane and moral considerations.

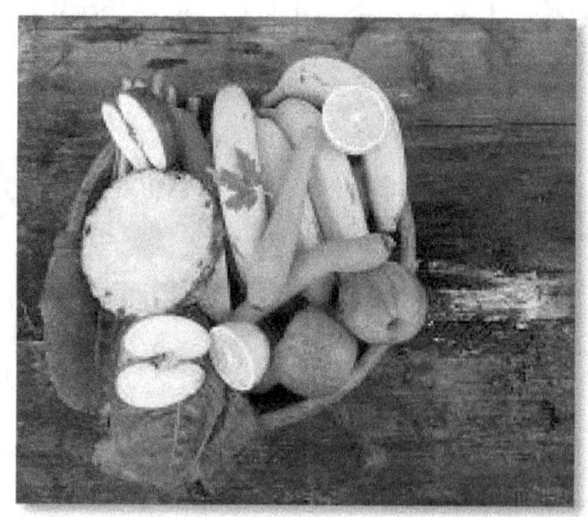

Veganism is to live in harmony with nature and the world around us, to understand ourselves as a part of this nature.

This also includes refusing fishing and hunting, a circus where animals work, and zoos, and everything else where there is at least a hint of unnatural treatment of animals.

Vegans absolutely exclude from the diet all products of animal origin, even seemingly innocent honey, since this is a product of exploitation. These people do not wear any fur products and clothes of all kinds of leather. Vegans use only cosmetics, the production of which did not use components of animal origin, as well as in the production process, which were not carried out on animals. Veganism is often called the extreme form of vegetarianism, although this is not entirely true. An extreme form of vegetarianism, rather, should be called a raw food diet.

RAW FOOD DIET

A raw food diet is a food system in which foods are consumed that did not go through any kind of heat treatment in the kitchen, such as stewing, baking, frying, smoke-dry, and others. It is believed that with this method of nutrition, the nutritional value of the products is fully preserved.

Raw foodists exclude from the diet of all products of animal origin and really eat exclusively raw vegetables and fruits. Food is never cooked. It is allowed to dry in the sun or in the oven at a temperature of no higher than 42 degrees. The list of allowed foods for raw foodists includes fresh fruits and vegetables, cereals, dried fruits, nuts, berries, herbs, germinate various cereal seeds and all kinds of cold-pressed oils.

FRUITARIANISM

Eating fruit is probably the sweetest type of raw food diet.

Fruitarians themselves define their diet as a diet with a predominant content of raw fruits in the diet (from 75 to 100% of the diet), sometimes with the addition of some other vegetarian foods (more often nuts and seeds, less

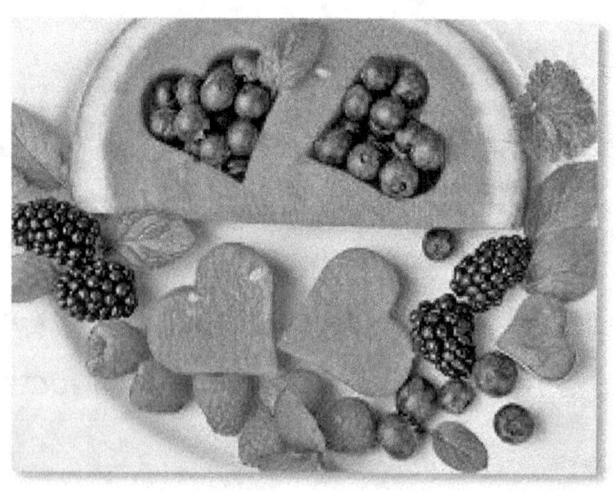

often some vegetables). Some of the strictest followers of the Fruitarian diet eat only those fruits and nuts that themselves fell from the trees, explaining this by the desire not to participate in the killing of any living creatures, including plants.

However, the balance of such a diet is subject to great doubt by well-known nutritionists.

Scientists from the University of Columbia (Columbia University in the City of New York) have proved that a fruitarian diet leads to a serious deficiency in the human body of substances such as zinc, most B vitamins (especially B12), protein, iron, vitamin D, calcium, and essential fatty acids.

Short-term dietary courses based on Fruitarianism can be considered as diet options for those who want to lose weight or seek to cleanse the body. But it should be remembered that even extreme diets, such as fruitarianism, can only be followed for a short time after consulting a nutritionist, and in the presence of any serious illnesses, only after consulting a doctor.

POLOTARIANISM

Polotarianism (pollotarianism) is an unusual type of vegetarian diet. This diet excludes the consumption of meat of animal type mammals (red meat). In this case, it is allowed to eat poultry meat, fish, eggs, milk.

PESCETARISM

Pescetarism - from the word pesce or pescado, which means "fish" - is an unusual type of vegetarian diet too. This diet allows you to eat fish and seafood. Dairy products and eggs usually are not consumed. However, 70-80% of the diet consists of vegetables, herbs, cereals, and legumes. Fish and seafood in the diet play only the role of an additional source of protein. A pescetarian diet is similar to a traditional Mediterranean diet. Like the Mediterranean diet, a healthy pescetarian diet consists of lots of fruits and vegetables, whole grains, nuts, and legumes. This diet is quite flexible. In addition, most pescetarians, like vegetarians, leave dairy products and eggs in their diets.

PLANT-BASED DIET VS VEGANISM VS VEGETARIANISM - WHAT'S THE DIFFERENCE?

Veganism vs Plant-based diet

A plant-based diet is based on plant-based foods and is virtually no different from a vegan diet in terms of nutrition. It's just a nutritional style of plant-based foods for maintaining and improving health.

Veganism is not only a plant-based diet but also a special ethical lifestyle. Strict veganism is to live in harmony with nature and the world, to protect all kinds of animals and stop any exploitation of creatures that live next to us on our planet. Most vegans decide to follow this diet for cultural, ethical, or religious reasons.

Vegans try to avoid all forms of cruelty too, and exploitation of animals for food, clothing, or any other purpose. This doesn't necessarily infer that vegans consume lots of wholefood meals, they can consume processed foods and snub their veggies. Just like anyone else, they can consume (vegan-friendly) gummy candy, potato chips and even cookies.

A plant-based diet, on the other hand, places more emphasis on consuming whole fruits and vegetables, eating lots of whole grains, and avoiding or minimizing the consumption of processed foods or animal products for health reasons. There are no definitions or strict guidelines for what makes up a plant-based diet other than placing emphasis on the consumption of fresh produce and eating a minimal quantity of processed foods.

Vegetarianism vs Plant-based diet

The main difference is that different types of vegetarians can eat some products of animal origin (milk, cheese, eggs, sometimes even fish or poultry). We talked about this in detail above. A plant-based diet consists solely of plant-based foods and focuses on the consumption of fresh produce and eating a minimal quantity of processed foods. And any products of animal origin are excluded.

Chapter 2.
Health Benefits

Of course, you should be familiar with this phrase, "You are what you eat" for a good reason: It has been used for over 250 years due to the concept that you are healthy and fit to eat healthy foods. Take it. The first literal use of the phrase came in 1923 when nutritionist Victor Lindelohr was quoted (surprisingly in beef propaganda): "Ninety percent of diseases known to man are caused by cheap food. You are the same. You are what you eat. "

To eliminate toxins

Almost a century later, we are still plagued by diseases that can be attributed to "cheap food" but also to chemicals, preservatives, antibiotics, pesticides, and even parasites in animal meat, humans. They consume a lot every year. To reduce the amount of artificial and harmful substances in their diet, over 60 million people around the world choose vegetarian. About 1 million of those who do not eat meat are vegetarians. In recent studies and surveys, the main reason why vegetarians * choose their lifestyle and diet "is to improve their overall health by choosing a natural approach to health."

By eliminating toxins associated with meat consumption, studies have shown that vegetarian and vegan diets can reduce the risk of cancer-related mortality by up to 50 percent while eating healthy foods, but this can slow progress. Delay or even stop.

HELPS AVOID OXIDATIVE STRESS

Oxidative stress in the body is another serious health problem that affects some consumers of animal products such as dairy and meat. One of the most harmful effects of eating meat in our body is that it causes the body's pH level to become too acidic, creating an environment in which bacteria and viruses can thrive, fatigue and discomfort can occur. Overall, it can affect a healthy person, and even cell damage may begin.

FLUSHES OUT URIC ACID

All foods we eat contain a natural ingredient called purine, which is essential for cellular health. Some products of animal origin (e.g., poultry, beef, pork, most seafood) have high levels of purine. When a lot of purine is consumed, our body metabolizes it as uric acid. Uric acid is naturally found in our body and is essential for a healthy body. For example, uric acid in our blood acts as an antioxidant and helps prevent blood vessels from being damaged. Therefore, the continuous supply of uric acid is essential to protect our blood vessels.

However, when we accumulate too much uric acid in our systems, we can cause problems like gout and kidney problems. Our kidneys have a job of keeping blood uric acid levels balanced, but a meat-rich diet can quickly increase them. When uric acid accumulates in our body, it crystallizes in what is called urinary crystals of monosodium. When these crystals accumulate, they can precipitate in organs such as the kidneys, causing painful inflammation in the joints, resulting in a condition called gout.

GIVES STRENGTH TO ENDURANCE ATHLETES

A plant-based diet is beneficial for endurance athletes (or for all others) because plants are easily digested by our bodies and can quickly supply the energy and nutrients in our bloodstream.

Quality sources of carbohydrates, proteins, and fats, plants are a great source of fuel for athletes who need to work on lean muscle health to maintain their full weight.

Less processing of flowers involved in plant uptake leads to optimal digestion before and after training when an athlete's body needs adequate nutrition to nourish or repair muscles without feeding excessive blood flow to the stomach. With serious animal meat

According to a 2006 study by the Committee on Medical Responsibility Physicians, another essential benefit of a vegetarian diet is that it is beneficial for weight loss as well as maintaining less body weight. The vegetable population is thinner than people who eat meat. They also experience lower rates of heart disease, diabetes, hypertension, and other life-threatening conditions related to overweight and obesity.

Endurance athletes always want to go faster and longer, and it's an efficient way to lose body fat. It's simple: The lighter you are, the quicker you'll be. To prove this point, look at Isaac Newton's second law of motion, which states that direct acceleration is by force and inversely proportional to mass. To illustrate this, here's an example: There are two runners A and B, 5 '10 "tall. Runner A weighs 150 pounds with 12% body fat, while runner B weighs 180 pounds. The body fat content is 25%. The muscles of both runners can produce the same amount of power. Runner A automatically works faster because the force generated by your muscles can make your body move more efficiently and with less effort. Overall it will be faster and more efficient Runner B will be slower because of the amount of power it generates to move more mass.

REDUCING THE IMPACT OF VEGETARIANS ON THE ENVIRONMENT

Being vegan can be more than what you eat. Many vegetarians also refuse to use products made from animal products. Most clothes you wear at this time are likely to have some animal products, even if you are not wearing leather or fur. Many colors, types of glue and materials are taken from animals. This is just another area to think about when you become a vegan. Being vegan and being aware of the environment usually go hand in hand. The production of meat and clothing causes a lot of pollution that is not contaminated in the world.

A 2012 article in Leather International magazine said: "The tanning industry is ranked fifth in the polluting industry by the New York-based Blacksmith and Green Cross. Leather is just a standard fabric that Americans and the rest of the world have. Consume on a mass scale.

The production of these commodities not only hurts animals but also hurts people who work in factories. Many third world countries, such as the United States, do not have environmental hardware controls. The yarn results in the inappropriate disposal of waste and other materials.

Exposure to the environment, as well as to people living near factories and beyond, damages the environment before removing the new leather jacket home, you have to go through the tanning process, tanning is the process of treating animals' skin to produce leather, which is more durable and less susceptible to decay after the skin is brown. Chromium sulfate is a common chemical in the commercial tanning industry. Used. According to a report, "The World's Worst Toxic Pollution Problems," Chromium puts at risk 1.8 million people worldwide.

Global warming has become a significant problem in recent years. Everyone, from our government to our grandparents, talks about it. With the world's population increasing daily, we need to produce more food. More than 70% of our grains grow in the United States. They are fed by animals that are slaughtered for meat. 16 pounds of grain is needed to produce a pound of meat! This system does not seem to be very efficient. If we were hungry, we would get 16 pounds of cereal every day for 1 pound of meat. According to a 2001 US Department of Agriculture report, "Today, the livestock population in the United States consumes more than 7 times the amount of grain consumed directly by the entire US population."

If nothing changes, hunger and malnutrition in the world will rise. The United Nations Food and Agriculture Organization (FAO) estimates that "925 million people in the world are always hungry". That's 13.6% of the estimated global population of 6.8 billion. Keep in mind that "hungry" does not mean that you eat a snack. "Hunger" is defined as "an uncomfortable or painful feeling of lack of food; a desire for appetite. It is also a state of exhaustion due to a lack of food." Most of you who have read this book have probably never experienced real hunger before the current system that we use to prepare food promotes desire all over the world.

Keeping a vegan diet is one way that can help reduce the global burden of our dependence on animal products. Vegetarianism is believed to be an expensive way to eat. Sure, if you eat all the alternative products it can be costly, but if you buy in bulk and prepare all your meals, it can be cheap. The reason meat and dairy are cheap is that the government subsidizes the industry. If the government did not support meat and dairy, it would not be able to provide them. "There are estimates that a hamburger will cost only $ 200," says Watch. It is not suitable for our body or for the world to make very cheap meat. Our government's massive subsidies on meat and dairy products affect countries around the world. According to Market Watch, the United Nations and other organizations report that agricultural subsidies in rich countries such as the United States reduce market prices, to the extent that developing countries in Africa and elsewhere are encouraged to import food. That local farmer can use. A more efficient way. "

HEALTH AND VEGAN

Many studies around the world have shown that a vegetarian diet is healthier and far less effective:

Prostate, ovarian, breast, and colon cancer: An 11-year German study found a 50% reduction in the risk of cancer by following a vegetarian diet.

Heart disease, hypertension, type 2 diabetes, and stroke - all of which are potentially reduced by eliminating red meat from a normal human diet. Studies have shown that just 3 ounces a day of unprocessed red meat can increase mortality rates by up to 13%. With processed meat (hot dogs, etc.) that add up to 20% to the balloon due to the concentration of nitrates and preservatives in those products.

Osteoporosis: Cornell researchers have found that people on a vegetarian diet help lower their risk of developing osteoporosis compared to people on a diet high in animal protein, including dairy. Even with the large amounts of calcium in dairy products, high levels of animal protein filter out more calcium from the bones consumed.

Many other health problems that we are not aware of yet: growth hormones, pesticides, antibiotics, preservatives and other unhealthy "substances" that have been deliberately added to animal products can have other side effects that We don't know them yet. Along with the spread of diseases that are contaminated in animal slaughterhouses (such as mad cow disease), participating in a very meat-based diet has the potential to have severe, undesirable and long-term health effects.

Chapter 3.
Vegetable Proteins and Amino Acids

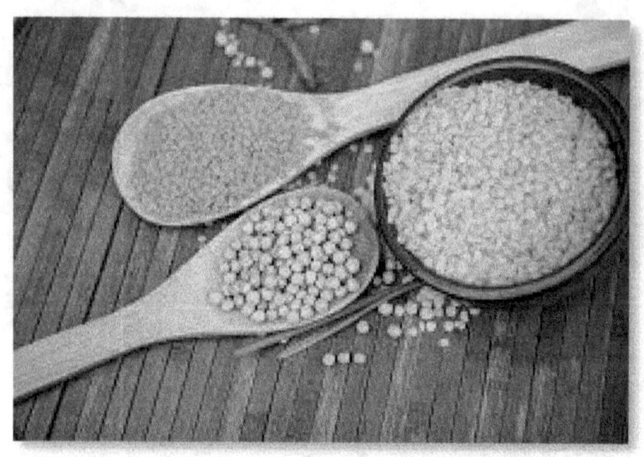

If you are going to stick to the vegan lifestyle, I think it is critical to explain why protein in your diet is crucial. Aside from water, protein is the second most found compound in your body. It is located in every part of your muscle, skin, tissue, etc. It is also within the healthy fats in your body, and these play a significant role in maintaining and keeping you healthy.

One of the most shared and well-known structures in our body that rely on protein is our muscles. Muscles are attached to the bone, thus allowing us to move and function daily. While this is most obvious, the organs in our body use internal muscles to make sure that we are working and ensuring every part is doing exactly what it was intended to. Even though several parts of our body are not made of protein, they tend to be held together by protein. This includes our nervous system, organs, and blood vessels. This should show you why protein is so important in our diet.

For one, if you want to follow a vegan diet, I'm actually going to show you that it is very possible, with all the recipes in this book! Second, if you go crazy and overload protein into your body, this can, in fact, affect your body in negative ways. Yes, there are issues if you don't have the needed amount, and yes there are issues if you take too much protein into your system. Finding the right healthy protein balance is an important thing to keep in mind when living the vegan lifestyle.

Additionally, consuming healthy protein can assist you in managing your weight since it takes longer to absorb a protein-rich meal. After taking in a meal with healthy protein, you are most likely to feel completely satisfied and full for much longer.

SHORTAGE

Unlike fat and sugar, our body has little ability to store healthy protein. Your body would undoubtedly begin to damage down muscular tissue if you were to quit consuming healthy protein.

Healthy protein shortage is uncommon in established nations, nevertheless, it can take place if you are not eating enough nutrient-dense food every day.

OVERCONSUMPTION

On the other side, it is feasible to consume excessive healthy protein. Some individuals think that excess healthy protein is secreted in pee; nonetheless, just part of the healthy protein is eliminated. An additional part of the healthy protein is transformed into sugar for power or saved as fat.

If you consume too much healthy protein – and several calories as an outcome – you run the risk of gaining weight from excess calorie intake.

You are most likely not obtaining adequate carb or fat for your body to work appropriately if your calorie objective remains on track however, you obtain even more healthy protein than you require. The trick to having correct nutrition is accomplishing the right equilibrium of macronutrients.

Consuming huge quantities of healthy protein can lead to dehydration in elite professional athletes. If you comply with a high healthy protein diet regimen, it is crucial to drink plenty of water.

EXCESS CONSUMPTION OF PROTEIN

It is entirely appropriate to boost the quantity of healthy protein you consume, yet, there are, obviously, restrictions to the amount you need to eat. According to the Harvard Medical School, consuming 2 grams of healthy protein per kg of body weight or even more could be poor for your wellness. Several of the downsides that can take place when eating way too much healthy protein consist of:

High cholesterol, commonly related to the intake of excessive hydrogenated fat, which is in animal-derived foods and various other edible items like coconuts.

Gastrointestinal system concerns, consisting of looseness of the bowels and irregular bowel movements.

Kidney troubles, consisting of kidney rocks and other kidney conditions.

Increased risks of age-related conditions, consisting of cardiovascular diseases and the formation of cancer cells.

WEIGHT GAIN.

Consuming huge quantities of healthy protein over a brief amount of time most likely will not impact you in these ways. Long-lasting adherence to a high-protein diet plan might adversely affect your wellness.

It is vital to make sure that you are still consuming a well-balanced diet regimen if you choose to take in a significant quantity of healthy protein each day. In this situation, that would certainly indicate picking various kinds of healthy protein, like fatty fish, eggs and plant-based proteins, in addition to animal-derived products. Taking in a range of healthy proteins will certainly assist enhance the number of nutrients in your diet regimen, decrease the quantity of hydrogenated fat you are eating and make you far better off about your total wellness.

CONSUMING TOO LITTLE PROTEIN

Taking in too little healthy protein is simply as bad as taking in too much over lengthy durations of time. Individuals that take in little quantities of healthy protein might merely by sticking to vegetarian, various other diets or vegan diet regimens that include many plant-based foods.

You must realize that a healthy protein consumption of less than 5 percent, can trigger loss of muscular tissue mass. It is thought that too little proteins in the system are insufficient to maintain a healthy living standard. Low-fat, low-protein, high-carbohydrate diet plans include eating a minimum of this much healthy protein.

Some individuals think that a high-protein diet plan can cause kidney damages and the weakening of bones. However, these claims are not sustained by scientific researches.

Healthy protein limitation is useful for individuals with pre-existing kidney problems, but healthy protein has never been revealed to trigger kidney damages in healthy and balanced individuals.

A higher intake of healthy protein consumption has been discovered to reduce blood pressure and assist in combating diabetes mellitus, which are two of the major threat variables for kidney illnesses. Anyway, any possible risks of people who adopt a healthy protein diet are debunked by all the favorable results generated by these elements.

Healthy protein has additionally been criticized for the weakening of bones, which appears weird if you think that there are researches that reveal that it can prevent and cure this problem.

Generally, there is no proof that a fairly high healthy protein consumption has any kind of negative impact on healthy and balanced individuals attempting to remain healthy and balanced.

Healthy protein does not have any kind of adverse impact on kidneys in healthy and balanced individuals, also, researches reveal that it brings enhanced benefits to bone wellness.

Here's a look at specific factors that impact your protein needs:

Because healthy protein isn't one-size-fits-all, there are particular groups that require even more and might have a more challenging time obtaining a sufficient amount of protein.

Excellent information for those giving up meat-based foods: if you are consuming sufficient calories, selecting a plant-based diet regimen does not immediately indicate you are not eating sufficient healthy protein. According to the Academy of Nutrition and Dietetics, the terms "full" and "insufficient" healthy protein are deceiving. "Protein from a selection of plant foods, consumed throughout the training course of a day, materials sufficient of all essential (necessary) amino acids when calorie needs are fulfilled," the Academy claimed in a 2016 placement declaration.

Vegans, and vegetarians, might require paying a little more focus to what foods provide to assure they get the very best protein-for-calorie worth. It is harder for them than ordinary meat-eaters. However, consuming a different diet plan that consists of protein-rich vegetables and soy will undoubtedly maintain your body and muscle mass just fine.

Healthy protein isn't simply an issue for the shake-guzzling bodybuilder intending to develop muscle - or the elite runner attempting to maintain it. Enough healthy protein is required in all degrees of physical fitness and the capacity to sustain the development of muscular tissue and functions as a foundation.

The IOM's standards were based upon research studies in inactive people. The American College of Sports Medicine, and the International Society of Sports Nutrition, suggest going for even more healthy protein if you are energetic, as much as 2 grams/kilogram of body weight daily to preserve muscular tissue mass. While maintaining healthy protein within 10 to 35 percent of your daily calories still is correct, professionals suggest eating 15 to 25 grams of healthy protein within an hour post-workout (an instance is 1 cup of milk, 1 ounce almonds and 5 dried out apricots) to optimize outcomes.

Does even more healthy protein equal far better outcomes? Not so, states an existing study, which recommends that advantages level off after suggested consumption. "It is kind of like including washing cleaning agent to your clothes - it is not going to get them cleaner - but having the correct amount, at the correct time, is essential," Crandall claims.

Foods high in a particular amino acid-the foundation of protein - called leucine - might be most reliable for the upkeep, repair work and the development of muscle mass. High-leucine foods are, for example, milk, soybeans, salmon, beef, hen, eggs and nuts like peanuts. While you need to aim to satisfy your healthy protein needs from food, whey healthy protein supplements are additionally high in leucine and are a research-backed alternative.

As we age, our bodies end up being much less effective at changing the healthy protein we eat into brand-new muscle mass. The outcome is steady muscular tissue loss that can cause lowered resilience, frailty and loss of movement. You can offer "Father Time" a one-two strike by keeping eating energetic and enough healthy protein-dense food.

Two worldwide study halls advise that older people should consume the same amount of proteins as young professional athletes: keep your minimum everyday healthy protein consumption to 1 gram/kilogram of body weight (68 grams and 80 grams for a 180-pound male and a 150-pound female, respectively).

They have expanded your protein intake - about 25 to 30 grams of healthy protein at each meal - since the quantity of healthy protein required to set off muscular tissue upkeep is greater. According to research published by the Journal of Clinical Nutrition, males and females aged 67 to 84 that consumed more healthy proteins and had more health benefits over 2 years resulted in having extra muscular tissue than those that failed.

"Protein requires to be increased by a minimum of 10 grams daily throughout the 3rd and 2nd trimesters because your infant is growing - and thus it requires the means to grow," states Rachel Brandeis MS, RDN, that concentrates on maternity nutrition. The IOM suggests that expecting ladies should consume a minimum of 1.1 grams/kilogram of body weight daily or around 70 grams in total.

The current study recommends that during the entire maternity period healthy protein requirements might be somewhat greater than these previous numbers, nonetheless, it is ideal to sign in with a physician or signed up dietitian to see just how much healthy protein is right for you.

When it comes to nursing mothers, your body will certainly require extra calories and healthy protein to produce an adequate amount of milk.

Healthy protein is a vital nutrient, and when you are consuming a diverse, healthy and balanced diet regimen, you are most likely obtaining an enough. Objective to consist of protein-rich foods throughout your day, not simply at supper. If you are an individual that requires even more protein - whether you are energetic, older or pregnant - you might need to be extra aware of your healthy protein consumption to make sure you are obtaining what you require.

Legumes, nuts, and seeds are excellent resources of healthy protein. Some veggies (such as spinach or kale) and grains (such as quinoa) additionally supply healthy protein in smaller percentages.

To maintain your healthy proteins from plant-derived food healthy and balanced, you should select recipes and cooking approaches that protect their 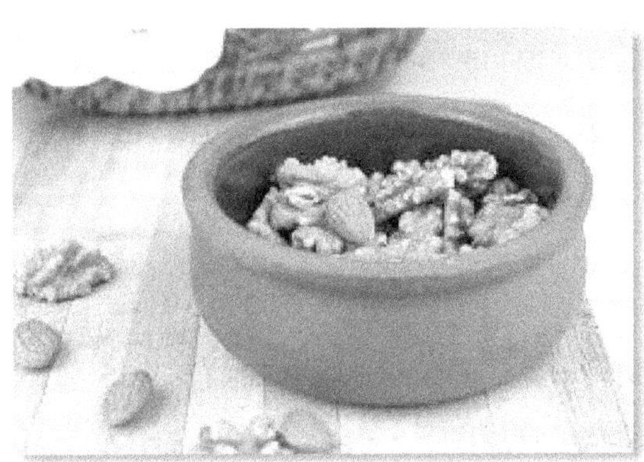 dietary advantages - using tofu as a substitute for meat in a stir-fry, including seeds or nuts to a supper salad, or making use of completely dry beans like kidney-shaped beans, navy or black beans as your essential healthy protein resource for a couple of dishes.

Why you must consume plant-based healthy protein

Healthy protein plays numerous crucial functions in the body, so it is essential to obtain a sufficient amount of them. (How much you require relies on your age, sex, task and weight.) Plant healthy protein can be an excellent choice in contrast to healthy animal protein. Below there are a couple of reasons that explain that.

PLANT HEALTHY PROTEINS ARE FULL, HEALTHY PROTEINS

There is a preferred false impression that healthy plant protein is substandard to healthy animal protein, yet, that is not the case. You do not need to consume meat to obtain ample quantities of healthy protein.

Healthy animal protein usually has more healthy protein per offering than vegetables. It is commonly thought to be a total healthy protein because it includes all the 9 necessary amino acids that our bodies cannot make by itself. Since we require to obtain them from our diet plan; our body produces the others that we need. These amino acids are called crucial. Numerous plant foods do not include all the 9 vital amino acids and are occasionally described as insufficient healthy protein.

Amino acids are the structure blocks of healthy protein, and in general, we require sufficient quantities for the body to operate. As long as we consume a range of foods over our days that jointly have all of the vital amino acids, the body has the raw product it requires to make healthy proteins.

That stated some plant foods are taken into consideration full, healthy proteins - spirulina, chia seeds and maca powder, among others.

PLANT HEALTHY PROTEIN IS A LOT MORE LASTING

When picking what to place in our mouths, we should take notice that environmental changes and the decreasing of all-natural sources make it much more essential than ever before to be careful of the wellness of the earth.

It is clear that our food system is a significant motorist of environment adjustment, air pollution, and the exhaustion of natural deposits - professionals have discovered that as much as 75 percent of complete farming exhausts originate from generating animal-based food. Without committed initiatives and technical steps to minimize this problem, our food system's effect will just become worse, making our atmosphere uninhabitable and risky.

On a serious notice, however, the future is not completely grim as we could expect - making the change towards much healthier, plant-based diet regimens is a vital component of the service. Healthy plant protein is extra effective and much less resource-intensive to generate than healthy animal protein, making it the premium option in terms of sustainability.

Plant healthy protein sustains healthiness

Healthy plant-derived protein tends to be high in vitamins, minerals, fiber, antioxidants and various other substances that we require to remain healthy and balanced. Some kinds include considerable quantities of healthy and balanced fats, as well. Beans, nuts, seeds and entire groups of grains are all healthy plant proteins that you should consume.

Research studies have revealed that healthy plant protein, as part of a plant-based diet plan, lowered the body weight and enhanced insulin resistance in obese individuals. If you are looking to reach your healthy and balanced weight, including even more plants to your diet plan is a terrific step, to begin with.

Extra research studies have established that plant-based diet plans might decrease high blood pressure, cholesterol levels and body mass index, and minimize the risk of stroke and cardiovascular diseases. In people with Type 2 diabetic issues, a plant-based diet plan has been discovered to assist the management of blood sugar levels. An added study has revealed that an extra plant-based diet regimen might reduce the risk of creating diabetic issues.

This is a piece of motivating information for individuals currently managing several of the following problems: patients being treated for persistent illness and heart problems that consume a plant-based diet plan might not require as numerous drugs. For healthy and balanced individuals, plant-based diet plans have been connected with a lowered danger of all-cause death amongst United States adults. Thinking about all the advantages, it is understandable why medical professionals and specialized nutritionists are suggesting a plant-based diet regimen to the majority of their clients.

PLANT HEALTHY PROTEIN IS KINDER TO ANIMALS

Ninety-five percent of stocks in the U.S. are elevated on agriculture, according to the ASPCA. These dismals, contaminated commercial ranches, created to fulfil the need for meat and various other animal-based foods, have brought on an unknown quantity of animal ruthlessness and suffering.

While an enhancing variety of meat and dairy products businesses are functioning to enhance problems for their animals, very little regulation remains in the area to maintain animals risk-free. There are no government regulations to secure animals on ranches, and states that have anti-cruelty regulations hardly ever implement them.

The straightforward truth of the issue is that consuming even more plants suggests (we would certainly assume) consuming fewer animal products, which is much better for your wellbeing, for the wellbeing of the earth, and definitely of the one of the animals.

PLANT HEALTHY PROTEIN IS AFFORDABLE

A plant-based diet plan does not need to cost a fortune. On the other hand, plant healthy protein can be unbelievably budget-friendly.

Peas, beans and lentils are one of the most inexpensive and most versatile, recipe-friendly resources of plant healthy protein. Various other choices that set you back a little bit, yet, are really high in healthy protein (seeds and nuts, as an example) can still be a good value, specifically if you purchase them wholesale. They additionally give high fats, together with various other essential nutrients, providing you much more value.

WAYS TO GET PROTEIN WHEN YOU'RE ON A PLANT-BASED DIET

Think it or not, you can really prosper, and never ever endure a healthy protein shortage on a plant-based diet. Since you should consider precisely how energetic your way of living is, a well-thought whole food plant-based diet regimen offers even more than sufficient healthy protein to please the body's demands without all the artery-clogging saturated fats that are present in the current American diet plan.

NOT ALL HEALTHY PROTEIN IS DEVELOPED EQUIVALENT

Healthy protein is composed of parts called amino acids. Throughout food digestion, your body will certainly break down the healthy protein right into these amino acids and will utilize them for various processes in your body. A few of these uses consist of constructing bones, muscle mass, and various other body cells, producing hormonal agents, and sustaining natural chemical features.

There are 22 amino acids, 9 of which your body cannot make, so they should be acquired from your diet plan. These are generally called vital amino acids.

Numerous plant-based healthy protein resources have some, yet not every one of the crucial amino acids. This makes it essential to consume a range of these vegetarian or vegan foods throughout the day.

Chapter 4.
Join Diet with Sport Activities.

Exercise is essential for health and eating healthy food will help you get the most out of the exercise that you do. Nutritional deficiencies and poor eating habits can impair performance. Here are a few great meals and snacks that you should consider adding in so that you will shine:

CARBOHYDRATES

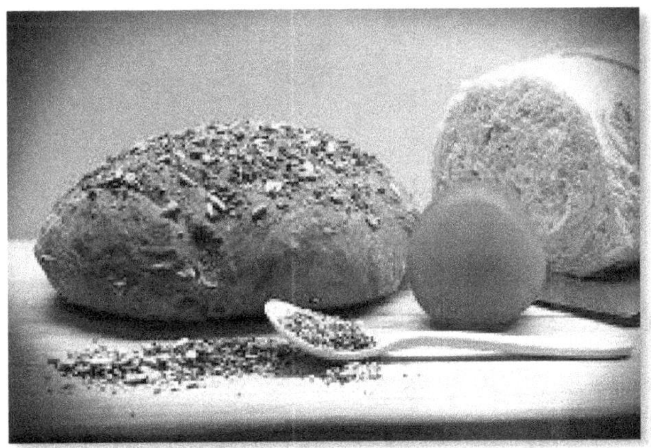

Usually, carbohydrates are the primary fuel, which is utilized when you are doing high-intensity exercise. The carbohydrate needs for athletes are close to those for anyone else on a per-calorie basis (a minimum of 55% of your total daily intake of calories). More specific recommendations for athletes are done based primarily on weight, and they range on average from 6-10 grams per kilo of body weight each day. A staggering amount of evidence shows that the availability of carbohydrates boosts performance and endurance. Excellent sources of carbohydrates include vegetables, fruits, and whole grain foods. Depending on how much exercise is done and how strenuous the workout is, carbohydrate synthesis peaks 30 minutes to 2 hours post activity. Foods that are rich in carbohydrates and which have a moderate to high Glycemic index offer an easily available source for the production of glycogens.

WATER

Maintaining the optimal state of hydration is essential so that any athlete can operate at peak performance levels and reduce the incidences of injury. Dehydration, which is defined as a body weight loss of more than 1% due to loss of fluids, results in a variety of symptoms, including dark urine with a strong odor, heat intolerance, fatigue, and headache.

More serious side effects include heat stroke, heat exhaustion, heat cramps, and neuromuscular fatigue. By maintaining a regular schedule of fluid consumption that equals at least eight 8-ounce glasses of water every day, symptoms like these are prevented easily. Fluid needs increase with an increased amount of exercise. Also, keep in mind that participating in activities at high temperatures, in low humidity, or at high altitudes can also increase your body's need for fluid replacement.

Follow these general guidelines to make sure that the hydration is never a problem:

- Drink 2 cups (or about 14 to 20 ounces) of fluid two hours before exercise.
- Drink 1 to 1.5 cups (or about 5 to 12 ounces) of fluid every 15 to 20 minutes during exercise.
- Drink 2 to 3 cups (or about 16 to 24 ounces) of fluid after exercising for every pound that has been lost during physical exertion. Weigh yourself before and after in order to determine how much fluid you are losing.

Water is the perfect fluid replacer, especially during activities which last less than one hour. For other more intensive activities that last longer than 60 to 90 minutes, electrolyte or carbohydrate-containing sports drinks may be useful both during and after exercise.

CALORIE AND PROTEIN REQUIREMENTS

A diet for the vegan athletes should take into account extra energy requirements above that of moderate level activity. The low-calorie density in many of the plant foods makes energy requirements become a major consideration.

During exercises, there is an increased protein breakdown and oxidation which is then followed by heightened muscle protein synthesis and further breakdown of proteins during recovery. The rise in the levels of circulating amino acids after one takes a protein-containing meal normally stimulates intramuscular protein synthesis in addition to slightly suppressing muscle breakdown of proteins.

Ingesting just carbohydrates into the body does not induce such increases in protein synthesis by the muscles. Furthermore, protein-containing meals have significant benefits to the immunity, muscle soreness as well as overall health as compared to carbohydrate-only meals.

Because of this, timing of protein content in meals is an important factor in recovery, muscle mass gain and maintenance.

The branched chain amino acids (BCAA) supplements; isoleucine, valine and leucine in a ratio of 1:1:2 have been specifically studied for their effects on muscle protein synthesis, performance and recovery. The oxidation of leucine supplements is significantly regulated during endurance exercises thus showing the necessity for increased intake of protein by athletes.

Research has suggested that the BCAA supplements do not affect performance significantly, but they attenuate exercise-induced muscle damages and also promote muscle protein synthesis. Plant proteins like sesame seeds, tofu, pumpkin seeds and sunflower seeds are great sources of BCAA supplements.

PROTEIN REQUIREMENTS FOR VEGAN ATHLETES

Every athlete (both vegan and non-vegan) require a greater protein quantity than sedentary individuals. Nevertheless, the amount of protein that is required has been a point of disagreement and confusion between the scientific community and the athletes. Proteins might comprise of 5 percent of the energy that is burned during exercises thus resulting in the need of positive nitrogen balance as raw material for the anabolic processes. This is to replace the losses and build any additional muscle mass. Insufficient ingestion of proteins leads to insufficient recovery and negative nitrogen balance.

POTENTIAL DANGERS OF EXCESS PROTEINS

There are no confirmed benefits for any athlete to consume over 200g protein. In fact, excess proteins usually have negative effects on the calcium stores, bone health, cardiovascular health and kidney function.

It is highly encouraged to use whole food protein sources like tofu, seeds, nuts and hemp seed meals which have been blended into smoothies and shakes.

It is important to note that isolated proteins powders are micronutrient-poor as compared to whole foods. Furthermore, their usage might pose health risks to individuals since excess animal proteins usually promotes cancers as a result of the increases in insulin growth factor 1-commonly referred to as IGF-1.

Animal proteins are not the only proteins which elevate IGF-1 levels but the isolated proteins from plant different plant sources also have a similar effect. The main factor which defines excess proteins for athletes is yet to be clearly defined due to the scarce studies on protein safety amongst athletes.

MUSCLE GROWTH

There is a big difference between maximizing health and maximizing muscle growth and body size. It is clear that a well-designed vegan diet will meet the nutritional demands of an agility and speed athlete like tennis, basketball, skiing, track and soccer. It used to be believed that is was not ideal maximizing muscle growth in larger athletes such as football linebackers or body builders. But there are modern techniques and vegan friendly supplements which can help.

Plant protein concentrates like maca, rice, hemp protein powders and pea are options whenever the athlete wishes to remain vegan or significantly reduce their dependency on the animal products while still supporting a high body mass.

In addition to promoting excellent health, an intelligently and carefully designed supplemented vegan diet will meet the caloric needs and supply enough protein to the body.

PICKING THE RIGHT FOODS

Learning what foods, you should choose, and how to make sure you get plenty of protein and calories, is what will help you jump on the plant-based bandwagon with easy. Before we start discussing foods and numbers, I want to divert for a second to a semi-related topic. I have used the terms plant-based and vegan interchangeably throughout this book, but I wanted to make sure you understand that it is possible for a person to be on a plant-based diet and not be vegan. If a person tells you they follow a plant-based diet, you can't be certain they eat vegan or not because plant-based diet could simply mean they incorporate more plant products and proteins into their diet, but they still consume some animal products.

I wanted to be clear, from this point on, the plant based I am talking about is a completely vegan diet. I am sure you already figured that out, but I want to let you know that just because somebody says plant-based does not necessarily mean vegan. This could save you at dinner parties in the future.

Now we can move into building a vegan diet for a bodybuilder. I am certain you already know this, but there are many different categories of bodybuilding. You have the traditional bodybuilding, and you also have physique, figure, and bikini. As a whole, no matter the type, bodybuilding will require a person to lose fat as well as put on muscle. Bodybuilders are able to do this through a combination of diet and strength training, and, by the time competition day rolls around, they are posing across the stage with a low body fat ratio.

But let's be real, building muscle is hard work no matter the diet you follow. And, if you are brand new to a plant-based lifestyle, supporting your athletic work with a vegan diet can be tough as well.

But it is possible, and easy, to slim down and bulk up while following a plant-based diet. It will require some nutrition strategies and proactive meal planning, just like competitive bodybuilding and smart vegan eating.

BODYBUILDING NUTRITION

If you are serious about being a vegan bodybuilding, you are going to have to have a good understanding of basic bodybuilding 'rules' for nutrition and food. The majority of bodybuilders, no matter what they eat, will split their season into two separate phases: bulking and cutting. With the bulking phase, they will consume a protein-rich and high-calorie diet, and they will strength train intensely to add as much muscle as they can. Then they will start the cutting phase. This is where they work to decrease their body fat, which usually done by slowly cutting down the fat and calorie intake.

These phases, both, will require the correct number of calories and the best balance of fats, proteins, and carbs. This is the trifecta of nutrients that will help you to drop weight, become stronger, and recover.

The actual breakdown of macronutrients for each person is going to be slightly different. The majority of bodybuilders will have a coach or nutritionist that they work with to help them figure out their macro and calorie needs in each phase. But there are some macro and calorie basics that you may find helpful, but we'll talk about that in a minute.

CALORIE INTAKE

While calorie counting is a touchy subject among many, some will argue that it is better that you do not do it, for bodybuilders, it plays a big part in their nutrition. When your goals are to add muscle mass, you have to make sure that your body has the fuel it needs to increase and build the size of the muscle fibers. And if you start reducing your calorie intake, you will start losing fat. This helps to make you look more muscular, even though you are not gaining new muscle.

You have to know what your true calorie needs are. You cannot guess, estimate, or assume things about your habits. You need to use real data that is based upon what you do and who you are.

Since not everybody is the same, you cannot give a baseline number for how many calories you need to consume. But lucky for you, there are a lot of online calculators that can do the math for you. Head over to bodybuilding.com and use their online calculator to figure out how many calories you should be aiming for during your different phases.

The numbers you get from these calculators should only be used as a starting point, and then you can start to experiment with those numbers to figure out what works best for you. The reason you have to play around with it is due to things like sleep quality, stress levels, hydration, metabolism, activity level, and menstrual cycle. They all affect the number of calories you need, just like muscle gain, loss, and maintenance.

This goes for vegan and omnivorous bodybuilders alike. Your daily calorie intake is not going to differ, no matter what diet you follow. Some like to think that vegans have to eat more calories, but that is simply not true.

Now, I know I just dangled an online calorie counter in front of your face, and you are free to use it, but you can also figure out some numbers on your own. Do not worry, though, it is not nearly as complicated as it may sound. You first have to start with figuring out your BMR, which is your basal metabolic rate with the Harris-Benedict equation. BMR is how many calories you expend through simply existing. This is based upon your weight, height, age, and gender. You can get your BMR using the calculator at globalrph.com.

Now you will take that number and combine it with your actual activity level. This is an additional movement other than just existing. This would include things like walking upstairs, going to the gym, running errands, or walking the dog. This will provide you with the approximate number of calories that you expend each day, which is considered your calorie needs. The calculator at globalrph.com takes this into consideration.

That means if you expend 2500 calories each day, you will have to eat 2500 calories to make sure that you maintain that weight. If you wanted to gain muscle, you are going to have to eat more than 2500 calories, which should come mostly from real plant foods. Mix that with some resistance weight training, and then you will be well on your way to more muscle.

While this may sound simple, implementing this into your life can be a struggle. But, trust me, it doesn't have to be that way. You simply need to focus on consuming healthy foods that you love along with enough calories, and you should not have a problem. To figure out the right foods for you, you also have to think about the nutrient density of them.

MACRO BREAKDOWN

A big mistake that people will make when they start following a vegan bodybuilding diet is that they forget to eat enough good calories, which can end up hurting the muscle-building goals. To make sure you are getting quality calories, you will need to know its macro breakdown.

Macronutrients, as mentioned before, are fat, carbohydrates, and protein. They are all major nutrients that your body has to have in order to function efficiently and properly. Counting your macros simply ensures that you consume a certain balance of each macro every day. Following a macro diet is also considered a flexible diet because you are allowed to consume whatever you want as long as you hit your numbers.

And guess what? This breakdown is the same for vegans and meat-eaters alike. The number of macronutrients you need to consume is going to remain the same. The only difference is you will use vegan foods to reach it. There are not any hard-and-fast rules as to what your macro breakdown needs to be, and your ratios will probably change depending on where competition day is sitting. For bodybuilders, you typically want to keep your carbs up, fats moderate, and protein high enough to help support the growth of muscle. Then you will typically cut that right before a competition by decreasing your carb intake a lot and your fat intake slightly.

For example, a general guideline breakdown ratio is 20/60/20 of fat, carb, and protein. This does not mean you have to follow those numbers exactly. You can play around with it and figure out which ratio works for you. Chances are if you have been a bodybuilder for a while, you already have a breakdown you have been following, and you can continue to follow that ratio.

VEGAN PROTEIN

There are a lot of different vegan protein sources out there, more than people know. You have hemp seeds, vital wheat gluten, fava beans, seitan, tempeh, bean pasta, textured vegetable protein, tofu, and lupini beans, just to name a few.

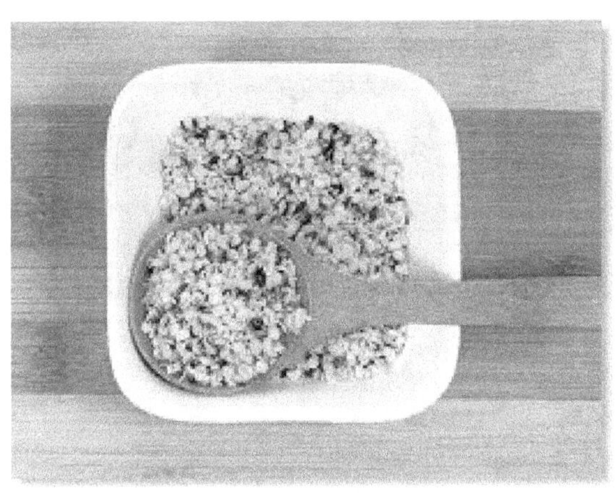

There is also vegan protein powder that you can use in place of whey protein in smoothies, and research has found that it is just as effective as whey protein. Oatmeal, black beans, kidney beans, nuts, nut butters, and amaranth are other great protein options for vegans. And there are even some foods that you wouldn't think contains protein that does, such as Brussels sprouts, mushrooms, chlorella, greens, and potatoes.

But it is also important to note that never single vegan protein option is created equal. Proteins contain amino acids. There are some amino acids, however, that are seen as "nonessential." This means that your body is able to make that particular amino acid on its own. There are some amino acids, though, that are "essential." This means that your body is unable to make it on its own without food.

There are nine essential amino acids that your body has to have in order to perform different functions, such as building muscles. Every animal protein source, such as fish, beef, eggs, dairy, pork, chicken, and turkey, contains all of these. When it comes to plant-based protein sources, they do not all contain all nine of these. But there are three exceptions: soy, buckwheat, and quinoa. Those three do contain all nine essential amino acids.

However, if you make a point of eating a variety of plant foods, your body will be able to store all of those amino acids and then combine them to create a complete protein. For example, beans and rice on their own are not complete proteins, but when you eat them both, they will provide you with all of the essential amino acids you need.

Keep Variety in Your Diet

When it comes to meal-prepping and counting calories and macros, it may be very tempting to eat the same things over and over again. But to make any meal plan good, whether you're vegan or not, is to make sure it has a lot of variety.

When you have variety in your diet, you will be getting all of the micronutrients you need, and you will be consuming all of the amino acids your body will need. This is especially true during your "cutting" period. This is when poor meal planning can end up causing nutritional deficiencies.

Yes, you can absolutely be a vegan bodybuilder while also gaining muscle and losing fat. And if you need a bit of inspiration, you can also turn to *Instagram* to see what others are doing.

Staples for Bulking Up

This is where we bring everything we have talked about together. When you weight the calories of a food against its nutrient density, and you factor in its macros, you will be setting yourself up for a muscle-building win. While you do want to make sure you get as many nutrients as you can, you cannot simply try to hit your calorie goals through kale alone.

So, where is the best place for you to start? The following five foods should be a staple in your kitchen when you want to bulk up.

- Bananas and other fruits
- Brown rice
- Lentils and beans
- Potatoes
- Oats

With different variations of these staples, you should be able to create a lot of variety and provide your body with lots of nutrition.

MIX IN AN EFFECTIVE EXERCISE PROGRAM

We have covered a lot on the nutrition portion of this chapter, but before you get the thought that you can gain muscle through food alone, you also have to have an effective exercise program. I am here to talk about food, so I will not get into this a lot, and hopefully, you already have an exercise routine. But I would like to share some fundamental pieces of information you should follow.

The foundation for your workout should be dumbbell and barbell exercises.

Do exercises that you like to do. Ultimately, if you are not having fun, then you are going to try to find a way to avoid doing it.

Have a workout plan that will target all of your major muscle groups, which includes abs, arms, shoulders, back, chest, and legs, to make sure that you stimulate growth in every around of your body and not just your biceps and chest. You can either choose to focus on one muscle group during your workouts, or you can mix up workouts to target it all of them.

The most important part is consistency. You have to put in enough time in order to get the results you want.

CREATE GOALS THAT YOU CAN REACH.

Document all of your workouts so that you can hold yourself accountable. You want to train consistently and keep a level of intensity that is going to elicit and ignite change.

It is important that you track your workouts along with your food. While this may seem like a waste of time, or super tedious, it will be worth it in the long run. Things will become second nature. And you may find that meal tracking is the secret to reaching all of your bodybuilding goals. You have the tools you need, so now you just have to do it.

Chapter 5.
Vegetarian Meal Plan for Bodybuilders

The freezer is one of the most useful devices when meal prepping but to make life easier, there are some things to keep in mind. It is a good idea to regularly clean out your freezer. Store your food at room temperature or in the refrigerator before freezing so that your food is not hot when you put it in-which thaws the ice and food around it.

Keeping the freezer full is more economical and air will be kept cold more easily but do not overload it so that no air can circulate. Be careful not to keep the door open for long when taking food in and out as the food inside will start to defrost and go bad.

BENEFITS OF MEAL PLANNING

There is one big benefit of meal prepping that prompts a lot of people to start doing it: you save a lot of time that you spend in the kitchen.

It allows you to save money.

Since you will think of each meal ahead of time, you will be able to plan it in a way that you can repeat some ingredients in several meals, which can end up saving you some bucks. Also, you'll naturally buy more friendly-freezer foods that can last a long time, so if you buy them in bulk, it ends up being cheaper in the long run. It will also stop you from eating out as much as you may have been, and your wallet will thank you for that.

It allows you to better control your portions.

Once again, because you will be prepping everything in advance. You will buy the exact quantities you need and have every meal already divided in different containers, so you can decide ahead of time how much food you will be consuming for each meal.

Save energy

Cooking a big batch of food at once uses up significantly less energy than cooking meals every single day.

Reduce waste

Food waste is a huge problem in today's society, but one way to reduce the wastage of food is through meal prepping. When you plan your meals, you will know how much food you need to cook and, therefore, you will buy only the ingredients you need. Thus, you will not have stocks of food items that do not get used past their best before date. Moreover, because you buy food in bulk, you reduce the amount of food packaging that gets thrown away.

It means one less reason to stress out.

You will not have to think about what you are going eat the whole week. Those times when you do not feel like cooking after a long day of work or when you do not have any ingredients to make a nice, healthy meal will not exist anymore.

It will reduce your food waste.

Since you know how much you will be consuming each week, you do not risk spending money on food that will end up getting rotten and going to waste. You can buy the exact quantities you need, which becomes even easier thanks to the recent trend of bulk grocery stores such as Costco and Trader Joe's.

WHAT MAKES A HEALTH MEAL PLAN?

The concept of meal prepping is pretty simple. The real challenge for some people comes when it is time to plan

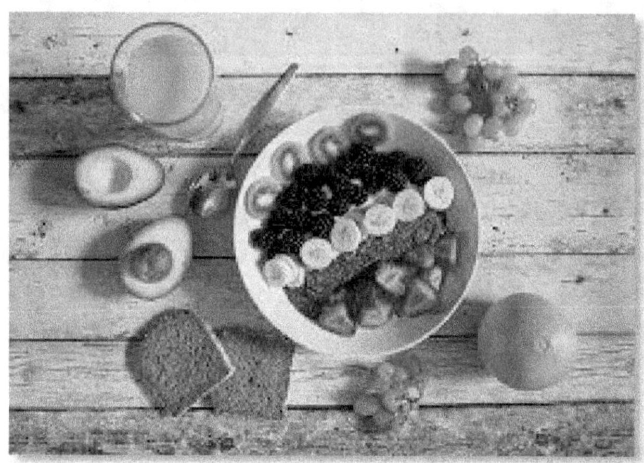

their meals for the week. In the beginning, this might take some time, but over time you'll understand what kinds of foods are good to include in your meal plans and making them will take less time.

A healthy vegan meal plan should:

- Avoid highly processed foods.
- Include fresh fruits and vegetables in every meal.
- Include whole grains instead of refined ones.
- Include a source of protein in every meal.
- Include low-sugar dairy alternatives.
- Include legumes, seeds and nuts.

- Incorporate fortified foods or supplements of vitamin B12, fish-free omega 3, and vitamin D (although you should speak to your nutritionist about this and get blood tests regularly to see if you need to adjust anything).
- Consist of a high variety of foods. A good tip for this is to make sure your pantry and fridge always look very colorful.

STORAGE, HEATING & FOOD SAFETY

This is one of the most important things to be informed about when it comes to meal prepping. You need to know how to store and heat each ingredient and meal that you prepare so that it doesn't rot before you get a chance to eat it. Otherwise, you risk wasting food that you spent money on or even getting food poisoning from eating food that went bad.

My advice is that you do your research each time you try meal prepping something new; it might take up some of your time at first, but with time you'll start getting a better understanding of how to store what.

Some general tips regarding food safety are:

- Prep meals for a maximum of one week.

- Keep the meals for three days in the fridge and freeze the rest. Unfreeze as time goes by.

- Stay away from plastic containers and opt for glass ones instead (*Otis Classic* and *Mcirco* are two great brands that do not break the bank). This will ensure that it is safe to reheat the meals in the microwave since there will be no risk BPAs getting into your food and, consequently, into your organism.

- For cooked meals, let them cool down before you put them in the fridge or freezer. Make sure not to leave them out of the cold for more than two hours after you are done cooking them.

- Always freeze your meals in airtight containers otherwise, your food can burn from the extreme cold and it will not be nice to eat.

- Always close your containers well because oxygen can make the meals good bad quicker.

- Keep foods that have a sauce away from the rest, otherwise everything will become soggy.

- Avoid defrosting your meals in the microwave as bacteria will become active and can even multiply. The best ways of defrosting food are by putting it in cold water and change the water regularly to ensure that it is always cold or by putting it in the fridge at least the night before but preferably 24 hours before you're going to eat it.

- Do not over-pack your fridge. It is important that air can circulate, so that it stays at a good temperature.

HOW TO SET UP YOUR KITCHEN FOR MEAL PLANNING

Something that makes meal prepping very easy is having the right tools in your kitchen. If you already have a well-equipped kitchen, you probably will not have to add a lot more supplies. If you are one of those people who has nothing more than the bare essentials, you might want to consider investing in some of the cooking material we are about to describe.

Some products are a bit more on the expensive side but know that you do not have to buy the best tools by the best brands ever. There are pretty affordable options for all the pieces of equipment that you need, and you can find them with a quick online research.

	Monday	Carbs g	Fat g	Protein g	kcal
Breakfast	Almond explosion 1 serving	29.5	15	25.4	355
A.m. snack	Hazelnut & chocolate bars 1 serving	21.3	14.2	20.6	296
Lunch	Lentil. Lemon and mushroom salad 2 servings	56.2	19.2	31.6	524
P.m. snack	Sunflower protein bars 1 serving	21.9	6.8	9.6	188
Dinner	Black bean and quinoa burgers 1 serving	40.5	10.6	9.5	200
	Total	169.4	65.8	96.7	1563

Tuesday		Carbs g	Fat g	Protein g	kcal
Breakfast	Powerhouse protein shake 1 serving	30	3.5	26.3	257
A.m. snack	No-bake almond-rice treats 1 serving	13.2	11.2	9.3	191
Lunch	Sweet potato and black bean protein salad 1 serving	48.8	14.5	11.4	370
P.m. snack	Overnight cookie dough oats 1 serving	22.7	11.3	30.7	316
Dinner	Stuffed indian eggplant 3 servings	54.9	18	13.2	435
Total		169.6	58.5	90.9	1569

Wednesday		Carbs g	Fat g	Protein g	kcal
Breakfast	Almond protein shake 1 serving	15.2	17	31.6	340
A.m. snack	Matcha energy balls 1 serving	21.3	21.2	14.6	335
Lunch	Southwest style salad 1 serving	51	16.8	11.2	397
P.m. snack	Lemon lime pie bars 1 serving	34.9	10.7	8.9	272
Dinner	Sweet potato sushi 1 serving	39.2	10.3	10.3	290
	Total	161.6	76	76.6	1634

Thursday		Carbs g	Fat g	Protein g	kcal
Breakfast	Cranberry protein shake 1 serving	19.9	16.8	23.6	325
A.m. snack	Mocha chocolate brownie bars 2 servings	34.6	7.6	54.6	416
Lunch	Cuban tempeh buddha bowl 1 serving	27.4	18.3	17.6	343
P.m. snack	Nutty blueberry snack squares 1 serving	21.7	13.1	10.3	246
Dinner	Tofu cacciatore 1 serving	33.7	9.5	13.6	274
	Total	137.3	65.3	119.7	1604

	Friday	Carbs g	Fat g	Protein g	kcal
Breakfast	Avocado-chia protein shake 1 serving	16.6	21.4	30.1	379
A.m. snack	Cranberry vanilla protein bars 1 serving	22.9	9.6	16.1	243
Lunch	Shaved brussel sprout salad 1 serving	45.3	18.7	11.5	396
P.m. snack	Spicy chickpea poppers 1 serving	21.5	7.8	9.1	192
Dinner	High protein black bean dip 1 serving	63	6.6	21.3	398
	Total	169.3	64.1	88.1	1608

WEEK 1: SHOPPING LIST

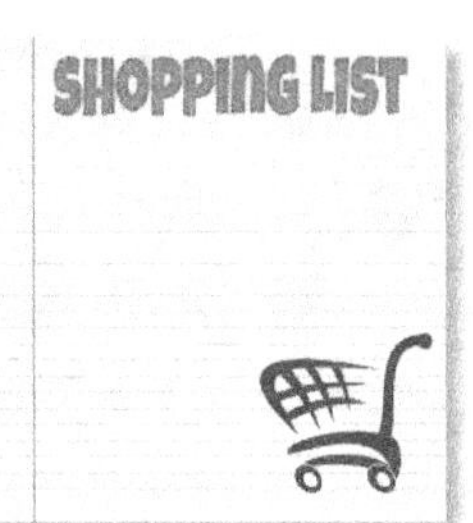

- 2 packages of unsweetened almond milk
- 1 package of oatmeal
- 1 package of raisins
- 1 package of almonds
- 1 package of peanut butter
- 1 package of vegan protein powder (vanilla flavor)
- 1 package of vegan protein powder (chocolate flavor)
- 1 package of hazelnuts
- 1 package of unsweetened cocoa powder
- 1 package of cashew butter
- 1 package of brown rice syrup
- 1 package of lentils
- 1 package of mushrooms
- 9 sweet or purple onions
- 1 bottle of extra virgin olive oil
- 1 package of garlic powder
- 1 package of chili flakes
- 1 lemon
- 1 package of cilantro
- 1 package of arugula
- 2 packages of oats

- 1 package of puffy rice cereal
- 1 bottle of maple syrup
- 1 package of sunflower butter
- 1 package of pure vanilla extract
- 1 package of cinnamon
- 1 package of nutmeg
- 1 package of salt
- 3 packages of black beans
- 1 package of quinoa
- 2 red bell peppers
- 2 green bell peppers
- 1 head of garlic
- 1 package of whole wheat flour
- 1 package of red pepper flakes
- 1 package of paprika powder
- 1 package of pepper
- 1 package of lettuce
- 2 green apples
- 1 pineapple
- 1 package of spinach
- 1 package of kale
- 1 package of spirulina
- 1 bottle of coconut water
- 1 package of unflavored vegan protein powder
- 1 package of almond butter

- 1 package of shredded coconut
- 1 sweet potato
- 1 package of cayenne
- 1 package of parsley
- 1 package of flaxseeds
- 6 japanese eggplants
- 3 roma tomatoes
- 2 packages of tomato paste
- 1 package of coconut sugar
- 1 package of cumin
- 1 package of turmeric
- 1 bottle of soy milk
- 1 package of coconut oil
- 1 package of raw cashews
- 1 package of pistachios
- 1 package of dates
- 1 package of matcha powder
- 1 package of gabanzo beans
- 1 package of mixed greens
- 7 cherry tomatoes
- 3 avocados
- 1 package of canned sweet kernel corn
- 1 package of chili powder
- 1 bottle of vinegar
- 1 package of chia seeds

- 1 package of pecans
- 1 package of sunflower seeds
- 2 packages of silken tofu
- 1 package of nori sheets
- 1 package of rice vinegar
- 1 package of agave nectar
- 1 package of amino acids, or tamari
- 1 package of cranberries
- 1 banana
- 1 package of hemp seeds
- 1 bottle of coconut milk
- 1 package of brewed coffee
- 1 package of basmati rice
- 1 package of tempeh, 14 ounce
- 1 package of dried blueberries
- 1 package of matchstick carrots
- 1 can of diced tomatoes, 28 ounce
- 1 package of balsamic vinegar
- 1 package of brown mustard
- 1 package of brussels sprouts
- 1 package of silvered almonds
- 1 package of walnuts
- 1 package of dried cranberries
- 2 cans of chickpeas
- 1 package of onion powder

WEEK 2: MEAL PLAN

Monday	Carbs g	Fat g	Protein g	kcal
Breakfast	Banana protein punch 1 serving	23.3	10	20.2	264
A.m. snack	Chocolate. Quinoa and zucchini muffins 1 serving	30.4	19.4	14.2	354
Lunch	Colorful protein power salad 1 serving	64.8	15.5	22.3	487
P.m. snack	Gluten-free energy crackers 1 serving	10.3	15.6	6.9	209
Dinner	Mango-tempeh wraps 1 serving	31.3	7.8	15.7	259
Total		160.1	68.3	79.3	1573

Tuesday		Carbs g	Fat g	Protein g	kcal
Breakfast	Almond protein shake 1 serving	15.2	17	31.6	340
A.m. snack	Sunflower protein bars 1 serving	21.9	6.8	9.6	188
Lunch	Creamy squash pizza 1 serving	62.5	8.6	18.4	401
P.m. snack	Chevy almond butter balls 1 serving	24.6	16.5	20.6	329
Dinner	Edamame and ginger citrus salad 1 serving	38.9	11.4	14.4	316
Total		163.1	60.3	94.6	1574

Wednesday		Carbs g	Fat g	Protein g	kcal
Breakfast	Cranberry protein shake 1 serving	19.9	16.8	23.6	325
A.m. snack	Overnight cookie dough oats 1 serving	22.7	11.3	30.7	316
Lunch	Super summer salad 1 serving	33.3	20.8	12.3	371
P.m. snack	Nutty blueberry snack squares 1 serving	21.7	13.1	10.3	246
Dinner	Sweet potato chili 2 servings	31.4	17	17.2	346
Total		129	79	94.1	1604

Thursday		Carbs g	Fat g	Protein g	kcal
Breakfast	Avocado-chia protein shake 1 serving	16.6	21.4	30.1	379
A.m. snack	Peanut butter and banana cookies 1 serving	20.2	11	10	220
Lunch	Vegan mushroom pho 1 serving	57.3	9.1	17.8	383
P.m. snack	Almond and date protein bars 1 serving	15.6	17.4	10.5	261
Dinner	Ruby red rootbeet burger 2 servings	46.4	9.8	11.2	318
Total		156.1	68.7	79.6	1561

Friday		Carbs g	Fat g	Protein g	kcal
Breakfast	Almond and date protein bars 1 serving	15.6	17.4	10.5	261
A.m. snack	Tropical protein smoothie 1 serving	44.4	6.7	27.9	350
Lunch	Lasagna fungo 1 serving	38	9.2	14.2	292
P.m. snack	Savory sweet lentil bites 1 serving	30.6	12.4	7.4	264
Dinner	Stacked n' spicy portobello burgers 1 serving	48.9	16	20.5	421
Total		177.5	61.7	80.5	1588

WEEK 2: SHOPPING LIST

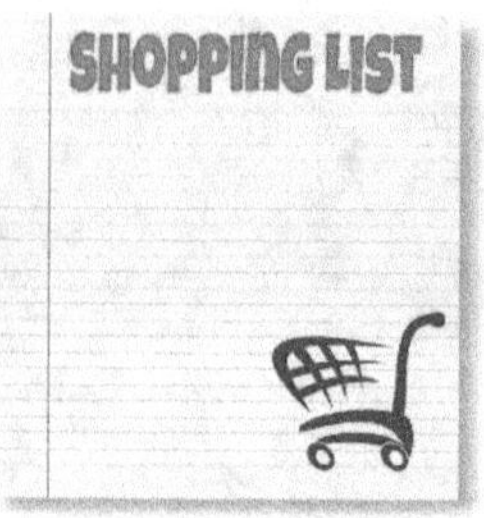

- 1 package of vegan protein powder, vanilla flavored
- 1 package of vegan protein powder, chocolate flavored
- 3 packages of almonds
- 1 bottle of oat milk
- 2 packages of quinoa
- 1 package of salt
- 1 package of pepper
- 1 package of coconut oil
- 1 package of olive oil
- 7 bananas
- 1 jar of applesauce
- 1 package of maple syrup
- 1 zucchini
- 1 package of dark vegan chocolate chips
- 1 bottle of almond milk
- 1 package of baking powder
- 1 package of cinnamon
- 1 package of nutmeg
- 1 package of vanilla extract
- 1 package of navy beans

- 1 package of green onions
- 1 head of garlic
- 1 package of green, or purple cabbage
- 1 package of kale
- 10 carrots
- 1 lemon
- 1 package of flax seeds
- 1 package of chia seeds
- 1 package of onion flakes
- 2 packages of peanuts
- 1 package of pumpkin seeds
- 2 packages of cashews
- 1 package of sesame seeds
- 1 package of paprika powder
- 2 packages of tempeh
- 1 package of sweet chili sauce
- 3 mangoes
- 1 package of lettuce
- 1 package of garlic powder
- 1 package of soy milk
- 1 package of cocoa powder
- 2 butternut squashes
- 1 package of red pepper flakes
- 1 package of oregano
- 1 package of cumin

- 1 package of paprika
- 1 green bell peppers
- 1 red bell peppers
- 1 package of broccoli
- 1 package of french lentils
- 1 purple onion
- 1 package of onion powder
- 1 package of carob chips
- 1 package of almond butter
- 1 package of pure vanilla extract
- 1 package of puffy rice cereal
- 3 avocados
- 1 package of mint
- 1 package of edamame
- 2 packages of green lentils
- 1 package of ginger
- 1 bottle of sesame oil
- 1 package of orange juice
- 1 lime
- 1 package of rolled oats
- 1 package of basil
- 1 package of red kidney beans
- 1 package of brussels sprouts
- 1 package of radishes
- 1 package of chickpeas

- 1 package of dried blueberries
- 1 package of sweet onions
- 1 can of diced tomatoes with green chilis
- 2 sweet potatoes
- 4 packages of extra firm tofu
- 1 package of cacao powder
- 1 package of coconut milk
- 1 package of peanut butter
- 1 package of cocoa nibs
- 1 package of mushrooms
- 1 package of hoisin sauce
- 1 package of gluten free rice noodles
- 1 package of raw beans sprouts
- 1 package of dried cranberries
- 2 large beets
- 1 package of gabanzo beans
- 1 package of balsamic vinegar
- 1 package of parsley
- 1 orange
- 1 package of blueberries
- 1 package of hemp seeds
- 1 package of lasagna noodles or sheets
- 1 package of hummus
- 1 package of nutritional yeast
- 1 package of allspice

- 1 package of sunflower seeds
- 1 package of portobello mushrooms
- 2 buns or wraps of choice
- 1 package of chili powder

Monday		Carbs g	Fat g	Protein g	kcal
Breakfast	Cinnamon apple protein smoothie 1 serving	21.7	10.3	48.5	373
A.m. snack	Lemon lime pie bars 1 serving	34.9	10.7	8.9	272
Lunch	Portobello burritos 2 servings	68	18.4	10.2	478
P.m. snack	Lentil radish salad 1 serving	25.3	10.7	12.4	247
Dinner	Mushroom madness stroganoff 1 serving	27.8	6.5	7.6	200
Total		177.7	56.6	87.6	1570

Tuesday		Carbs g	Fat g	Protein g	kcal
Breakfast	Candied protein trail mix 1 serving	19.5	28	14	387
A.m. snack	High protein cake batter smoothie 1 serving	27.2	7.6	16	241
Lunch	Creamy squash pizza 1 serving	62.5	8.6	18.4	401
P.m. snack	Chocolate .quinoa and zucchini muffins 1 serving	304	19.4	14.2	354
Dinner	Sweet and sour tofu 1 serving	24.3	11.5	8.8	236
Total		437.5	75.1	71.4	1619

Wednesday		Carbs g	Fat g	Protein g	kcal
Breakfast	Chewy almond butter balls 1 serving	24.6	16.5	20.6	329
A.m. snack	Gluten free energy crackers 1 serving	10.3	15.6	6.9	209
Lunch	Moroccan eggplant stew 1 serving	80.5	2.7	17.7	417
P.m. snack	Mocha chocolate brownie bars 1 serving	17.3	3.8	27.3	213
Dinner	Taco tempeh salad 1 serving	36.3	23	22.4	441
	Total	169	61.6	94.9	1609

Thursday		Carbs g	Fat g	Protein g	kcal
Breakfast	Banana protein punch 1 serving	23.3	10	20.2	264
A.m. snack	Sunflower protein bars 1 serving	21.9	6.8	9.6	188
Lunch	Refined ratatouille 1 serving	61.2	24.3	23.7	558
P.m. snack	Spicy chickpea poppers 1 serving	21.5	7.8	9.1	192
Dinner	Barbecued greens and grits 1 serving	39.3	17.6	19.7	394
Total		167.2	66.5	82.3	1596

Friday		**Carbs g**	**Fat g**	**Protein g**	**kcal**
Breakfast	Avocado chia protein shake 1 serving	16.6	21.4	30.1	379
A.m. snack	Cranberry vanilla protein bars 1 serving	22.9	9.6	16.1	243
Lunch	Roasted almond protein salad 2 servings	50	14.8	20	412
P.m. snack	Lemon lime pie bars 1 serving	34.9	10.7	8.9	272
Dinner	Sweet potato quesadillas 1 serving	54.8	7.5	10.6	329
Total		179.2	64	85.7	1635

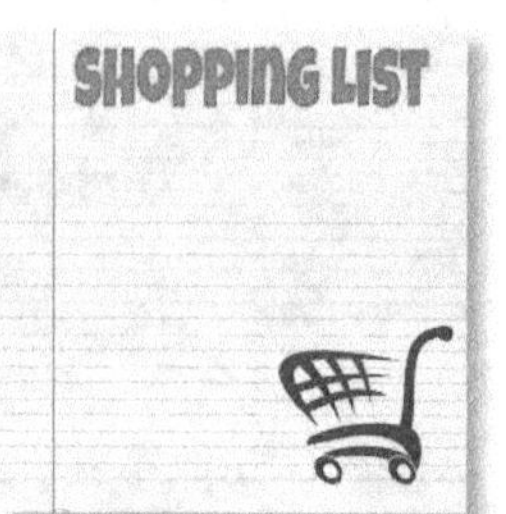

- 1 green apple
- 2 packages of coconut milk
- 1 package of cinnamon
- 1 package of salt
- 1 package of pepper
- 1 package of vegan protein powder, vanilla flavored
- 1 package of vegan protein powder, chocolate flavored
- 1 bottle of olive oil
- 1 package of coconut oil
- 2 packages of chia seeds
- 2 packages of pecans
- 2 packages of raw cashews
- 1 package of dates
- 2 lemons
- 1 package of portobello mushrooms
- 2 potatoes
- 3 avocados
- 1 package of cilantro
- 1 package of tomatoes
- 1 red onion

- 1 jalapeno
- 1 package of whole wheat flour
- 1 bottle of maple syrup
- 1 package of miso paste, yellow or white
- 1 package of sesame oil
- 1 package of chickpeas
- 1 package of green or brown lentils
- 1 package of silken tofu
- 2 radishes
- 3 cherry tomatoes
- 1 package of sesame seeds
- 1 package of gluten-free noodles
- 1 package of almond flour
- 1 package of tamari sauce
- 1 package of tomato paste
- 1 package of mushrooms
- 1 package of thyme
- 2 packages of spinach
- 1 bottle of apple cider vinegar
- 3 packages of almonds
- 2 packages of walnuts
- 1 package of nutmeg
- 1 package of cashew butter
- 5 bananas
- 2 packages of oats

- 1 package of pure vanilla extract
- 1 package of almond milk
- 2 butternut squashes
- 1 package of broccoli
- 1 package of french green lentils
- 1 head of garlic
- 1 package of onion powder
- 1 package of cumin
- 1 package of paprika
- 1 package of oregano
- 1 package of red pepper flakes
- 2 purple onions
- 1 jar of applesauce
- 1 package of baking powder
- 2 zucchinis
- 2 packages of quinoa
- 1 pineapple
- 1 ginger root
- 2 white onions
- 2 green bell peppers
- 1 red bell peppers
- 1 bottle of rice vinegar
- 1 package of low sodium soy sauce
- 2 packages of extra firm tofu, drained
- 1 package of cornstarch

- 1 package of coconut sugar
- 1 package of carob chips
- 1 package of puffy rice cereal
- 1 package of almond butter
- 1 package of flaxseeds
- 1 package of onion flakes
- 1 package of peanuts
- 1 package of garbanzo beans
- 1 package of golden raisins
- 1 package of turmeric
- 2 eggplants, large
- 1 package of allspice
- 1 package of green lentils
- 1 package of tomato sauce
- 1 package of sweet onions
- 1 package cocoa powder
- 1 package of agave nectar
- 1 package of brewed coffee
- 1 package of black beans
- 2 packages of tempeh
- 1 jalapeno
- 1 lime
- 1 large bunch of kale
- 1 package of oat milk
- 1 package of sunflower butter

- 2 heirloom tomatoes
- 1 package of fennel seeds
- 1 yellow squash
- 1 package of basil
- 2 cans of chickpeas
- 1 package of garlic powder
- 1 package of cayenne
- 1 package of collard greens
- 1 package of gluten-free grits
- 1 package of smoked paprika
- 1 package of peanut butter
- 1 package of shredded coconut
- 1 package of dried cranberries
- 1 package of navy beans
- 1 package of rice, of choice
- 1 sweet potato

Monday		Carbs g	Fat g	Protein g	kcal
Breakfast	Cinnamon apple protein smoothie 1 serving	21.7	10.3	48.5	373
A.m. snack	Nutty blueberry snack squares 1 serving	21.7	13.1	10.3	246
Lunch	Stuffed indian eggplant 3 servings	54.9	18	13.2	435
P.m. snack	Savory sweet lentil bites 1 serving	30.6	12.4	7.4	264
Dinner	Teriyaki tofu wraps 1 serving	20.5	15.4	12.1	259
Total		149.4	69.2	91.5	1577

Tuesday		Carbs g	Fat g	Protein g	kcal
Breakfast	Mocha chocolate brownie bars 1 serving	17.3	3.8	27.3	213
A.m. snack	Overnight cookie dough oats 1 serving	22.7	11.3	30.7	316
Lunch	Satay tempeh with cauliflower rice 1 serving	31.7	33	27.6	531
P.m. snack	Banana protein punch 1 serving	23.3	10	20.2	264
Dinner	Tex-mex tofu and beans 1 serving	27.8	14	12.7	315
Total		122.8	72.1	118.5	1639

Wednesday		Carbs g	Fat g	Protein g	kcal
Breakfast	Almond explosion 1 serving	29.5	15	25.4	355
A.m. snack	Matcha energy balls 1 serving	21.3	21.2	14.6	335
Lunch	Stuffed sweet potatoes 1 serving	55.7	17.1	20.7	498
P.m. snack	Sunflower protein bars 1 serving	21.9	6.8	9.6	188
Dinner	Red beans and rice 1 serving	32.3	8.3	7.9	235
	Total	160.7	68.4	78.2	1611

Thursday		Carbs g	Fat g	Protein g	kcal
Breakfast	Cranberry protein shake 1 serving	19.9	16.8	23.6	325
A.m. snack	Hazelnut and chocolate protein bars 1 serving	21.3	14.2	20.6	296
Lunch	Coconut tofu curry 1 serving	38.7	23	21.8	449
P.m. snack	Almond and date protein bars 1 serving	15.6	17.4	10.5	261
Dinner	Tahini falafels 1 serving	28	7.3	10.5	220
Total		123.5	78.7	87	1551

Friday		Carbs g	Fat g	Protein g	kcal
Breakfast	Almond and protein shake 1 serving	15.2	17	31.6	340
A.m. snack	Gluten-free energy crackers 1 serving	10.3	15.6	6.9	209
Lunch	High protein black bean dip 1 serving	63	6.6	21.3	398
P.m. snack	Lemon lime pie bars 1 serving	34.9	10.7	8.9	272
Dinner	Baked enchilada bowls 1 serving	34.6	27.1	15.6	417
	Total	158	77	84.3	1636

WEEK 4: SHOPPING LIST

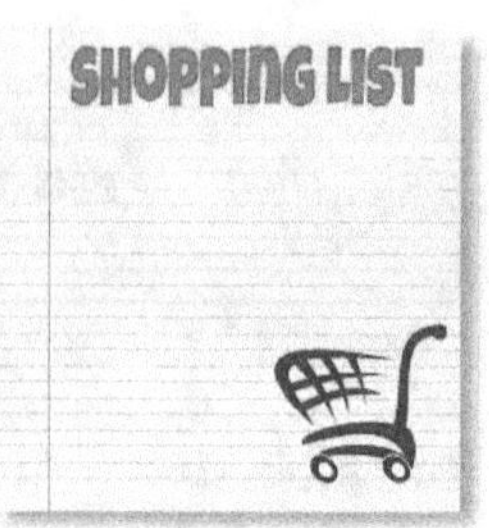

- 2 packages of coconut milk
- 1 package of cinnamon
- 1 package of vegan protein powder, vanilla flavored
- 1 package of vegan protein powder, chocolate flavored
- 1 green apple
- 2 packages of almonds, 1 raw
- 4 packages of cashews, 2 raw
- 1 package of puffy rice cereals
- 1 bottle of maple syrup
- 1 package of dried blueberries
- 1 package of salt
- 1 package of pepper
- 3 packages of black beans
- 6 japanese eggplants
- 3 roma tomatoes
- 3 purple onions
- 1 package of spinach
- 1 bottle of olive oil
- 1 head of garlic
- 1 package of tomato paste

- 1 package of coconut sugar
- 1 package of cumin
- 1 package of turmeric
- 5 green bell peppers
- 1 package of green or brown lentils
- 1 package of coconut oil
- 1 package of allspice
- 1 package of sunflower seeds
- 1 package of shredded coconut
- 1 package of almond butter
- 1 white onion
- 1 bottle of soy sauce
- 1 bottle of sesame oil
- 1 package of lettuce
- 1 package of sesame seeds
- 1 pineapple
- 2 packages of extra firm tofu
- 1 package of cocoa powder
- 2 packages of oats
- 1 package of nutmeg
- 1 package of pure vanilla extract
- 1 package of brewed coffee
- 1 package of agave nectar
- 2 packages of almond milk
- 1 package of flaxseeds

- 1 package of peanut butter
- 1 package of peanut butter
- 1 ginger root
- 1 bottle of rice vinegar
- 1 package of red pepper flakes
- 2 packages of tempeh
- 1 package of cauliflower rice
- 1 package of purple cabbage
- 1 package of oat milk
- 3 bananas
- 1 package of brown rice
- 1 package of tofu
- 1 avocado
- 1 package of paprika
- 1 package of chili powder
- 2 lemons
- 1 package of raisins
- 1 package of dates
- 1 package of hazelnuts
- 1 package of matcha powder
- 1 package of pistachios
- 1 package of sunflower butter
- 1 package of red beans
- 1 package of cauliflower
- 1 package of basil

- 1 package of parsley flakes
- 1 package of celery ribs
- 1 package of cranberries
- 1 package of chia seeds
- 1 package of hemp seeds
- 1 bottle of brown rice syrup
- 1 package of cashew butter
- 1 package of curry powder
- 1 package of turmeric
- 1 package of peas
- 1 can of fat reduced coconut milk
- 2 tomatoes
- 1 jar of applesauce
- 1 package of dried cranberries
- 1 package of chickpeas
- 1 package of tahini
- 1 package of broccoli
- 1 package of soy milk
- 1 package of onion flakes
- 1 package of pumpkin seeds
- 1 package of onion powder
- 1 package of pecans
- 1 sweet potato, large
- 1 bottle of mct oil
- 1 package of oregano

- 1 package of whole wheat flour
- 1 bottle of apple vinegar
- 1 package of nutritional yeast

Chapter 6.
How Many Macro Should I Eat?

Macronutrients or "macros" is the name given to three groups of energy-dense nutrients that make up the most basic components of our diets: carbohydrates, fats, and proteins. In addition to acting as fuel, they facilitate many of our bodies' functions and are broken down by our digestive system for use in bodily structures. Each macronutrient provides us with the following number of calories:

- 1 g protein = 4 calories
- 1 g carb = 4 calories
- 1 g fat = 9 calories

HOW DO YOU CALCULATE YOUR DAILY CALORIC INTAKE?

When preparing your meals, you will need to calculate two things: the macronutrients and the number of calories present in each meal. The recipes in this book take that responsibility off your shoulders; the included meal plan provides nutritional information for each day, with the correct balance of macronutrients and several options for different daily caloric intakes.

To benefit from the provided nutrition information, you need to know how much you need to eat in general each day. That is why we calculate daily caloric needs, also known as basal metabolic rate. This is essential for setting the bar for and keeping track of your daily macro intake. How to calculate your specific caloric needs is explained below:

- This is the formula you need to use to calculate basal metabolic rate (BMR):
- Men: BMR = (9.99 x weight in kilograms) + (6.25 x height in centimeters) - 4.92 x age in years + 5.
- Women: BMR = (9.99 x weight in kilograms) + (6.25 x height in centimeters) - (4.92 x age in years) - 161.

Multiply the BMR number with the activity factor that fits your lifestyle. With no exercise, your activity factor is 1.2. If you exercise one to three times a week, your activity factor is 1.375. If you engage in exercise three to five times per week, the activity factor is 1.55. For heavy exercise, six to seven times a week, the activity factor is 1.725. For athletes or those with heavy training sessions and/or a physically demanding job, your activity factor is 1.9. The number derived from this second calculation is the number of calories (kcal) required for maintaining a healthy weight.

Lowering your carb and fat intakes will allow you to burn fat more efficiently. For some athletes, a carb to protein to fat intake ratio of 50:25:25 is ideal. Once you have achieved your goals and wish to simply maintain your body weight, you want to focus on stabilizing your caloric intake with at least 15-20% of your calories coming from protein.

The following is a breakdown of how to achieve the 50:25:25 ratio on a 2000-calorie diet:

- 50% carbohydrates: 2000 x 50% = 1000 calories per day. To determine the amount needed, divide 1000 by 4 to get 250 grams of carbohydrates required daily.
- 25% protein: 2000 x 25% = 500 calories per day. Divide 500 calories by 4 to get 125 g of protein needed daily.
- 25% fat: 2000 x 25% = 500 calories per day. Divide 500 calories by 9 to get ~55.6 g of fat needed daily.

Tracking

Sticking to a meal plan and taking the time necessary to prep your meals will make the consumption of the proper number of daily macronutrients virtually effortless. By keeping a close eye on your carbohydrate, protein, and fat intake, your fitness goals will be within reach. Consciously tracking macros also makes it very easy to adjust your meal plan to address changing fitness goals and your body's needs.

Once you have a clear understanding of your daily calorie requirements, you can use this number to calculate the recommended number of daily macronutrients. As explained before, calories determine weight gain, loss, or maintenance. By consuming the correct ratios of macronutrients, you'll guarantee recovery and, combined with proper training, improve and optimize your muscular system and body composition.

Tracking macronutrients in this day and age is super simple thanks to apps like *MyFitnessPal* (https://www.myfitnesspal.com) and *MacroTrak* (iTunes) – (https://itunes.apple.com/us/app/macrotrak-macro-tracker/id1175925585?mt=8). If you do not have access to a smartphone or prefer a traditional or different method, tracking your intake by hand with a notepad or (digital) spreadsheet will work just fine.

Tracking effortlessly

The 30-day meal plan in this book further simplifies tracking calories. You only need to stick to the serving amounts of the recipes listed for each day, which eliminates the task of weighing portions. This meal plan covers a wide range of daily macronutrient targets so that you can plan for daily consumption of 1600, 1800, 2000, 2500 or 3000 calories, depending on your goals. Use this plan to your advantage!

The total number of macros you need to consume to reach your goals is based on your length, weight, and desired outcomes. The daily calorie sums in the included meal plan, that is designed to appeal to a wide audience, are made up of roughly 30-35% protein, 35-40% of carbs, and 20-25% fats.

You can mix and match the daily plans to create a variety of week- or month-long plans easily without the need for recalculation. The only time you will need to record calories and macronutrients is when you eat something that is not part of your meal plan.

Whether you are trying to lose weight, maintain it, or gain muscle mass, the meal plan can be rearranged to align with your desired outcomes.

Micronutrients such as vitamins, minerals, and electrolytes are the other type of nutrients that human body requires, but in comparison to macros, micros are required in much smaller amounts.

Except for fad diets, the human body needs all three macronutrients and cutting out any of the macronutrients puts the risk of nutrient deficiencies and illness on human health.

Carbohydrates that you eat is a source of quick energy, they are transformed into glucose or commonly known as sugar, and are either used right after generated or stored as glycogen for later use.

Protein is there to help with growth, injury repair, muscle formation, and protection against infections. Proteins are the compounds that are built from amino acids, which appear to be the building material for the creation of tissues in the human body. And our body needs 20 various amino acids, 9 of which cannot be produced by our body, and thus must be received from outside sources.

Dietary fat is another essential macronutrient that is responsible for many essential tasks like absorbing the fat-soluble vitamins (A, D, E and K), insulating body during cold weather, surviving long periods without food, protecting organs, supporting cell growth and inducing hormone production.

Usually, to stay healthy, lose weight and for some other reasons we are told to count the number of calories that we intake entirely, forgetting to tell to track macronutrient intake. Calculating and monitoring macronutrient intake can help not only with making health better and reaching fitness goals but can also help you understand which types of foods improve your performance and which are bad for you. If you would like to get such a calculator, you can type in a Google search, and there you will get lots of information on the topic.

Macronutrients are the food classifications that give you the power to bring out our fundamental human features, and they are boiled down right into 3 groups; healthy protein, fats, and carbs. When you recognize precisely how to determine your macros, it is simple to figure out just how much calories you are placing in your body every day and just how much energy you require to burn off the extra calories.

When most people hear about the vegan diet, they assume that vegans just eat a bunch of fruits and vegetables. And sure, most vegans do consume a decent amount of produce, but everyone should as they contain vital nutrients. You already know about your meals needing to contain fruits and vegetables to be balanced and healthy, you have heard that your whole life. Therefore, in this chapter, we will focus largely on other aspects that will help you to create healthy and balanced meals.

Many people new to the vegan diet worry about their ability to consume all the vital nutrients for human health. As a handful of nutrients are widely found in animal-based foods, they worry about losing health and developing life-threatening vitamin and mineral deficiencies. Thankfully, there are plenty of options for consuming a healthy and balanced vegan diet, which includes all the vitamins and minerals humans require for good health. In this chapter, you will learn about how to create these balanced meals that will ensure you consume all these needed nutrients.

NON-STARCHY VEGETABLES

While starchy vegetables, such as potatoes, have their place on the vegan diet, be sure that you include an abundance of non-starchy vegetables, as well. These vegetables have an abundance of both nutrients and fiber and are also much lower in carbohydrates and calories than their starchy companions.

HEALTHY FATS

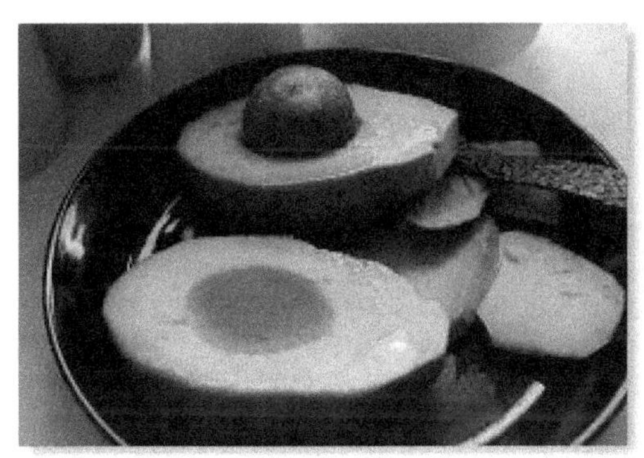

The low-fat dieting fad of the 1980s-90s couldn't have been more wrong. Consuming fat does not make a person fat. In fact, you need to consume fat in order to burn your body fat. Not only that, but fat is an essential nutrient to the human body that we must consume through our everyday diet.

However, not all fats are created equal. You should focus on monounsaturated fats such as those found in olive oil and avocados along with polyunsaturated fats found in walnuts and flaxseeds. While coconut oil does have many health benefits, this type of fat should be consumed in moderation as it is full of saturated fats. Thankfully, saturated fats are largely found in animal-based ingredients, and on a vegan diet, you will naturally consume lower levels of saturated fats. This, in turn, will improve your cholesterol and heart health.

Along with using these healthy fats in your meals, you can also add a drizzle of olive oil over a meal that might be light in fat or serve it alongside a half an avocado.

PLANT-BASED PROTEINS

Another large concern people have regarding the vegan diet prior to start is how they will get enough protein. Believe it or not, you get protein in many more sources than you might realize. For instance, whole grains have a decent amount of protein.

There are nine essential amino acids, otherwise known as the building blocks of protein, that humans require. The goal is to consume an enough all nine essential amino acids to create what is known as a complete protein. Soy products, such as tofu and tempeh, are a natural source of complete protein, whereas there are other ingredients you can combine to create a complete protein. For instance, when you consume beans and rice together, you create a complete source of all the essential amino acids.

You don't need to consume a lot of pre-made vegan meat replacements that you can find on the freezer aisle. While these can be helpful to use in creating last-minute meals or when you have a craving, they tend to be expensive and can easily be replaced with whole foods.

Some great examples of vegan whole food vegan protein include:

- Lentils
- Beans and Chickpeas
- Tofu and Tempeh
- Seitan
- Quinoa
- Amaranth
- Chia Seeds
- Flaxseeds
- Sesame Seeds
- Sunflower and Pumpkin Seeds
- Nuts
- Oats, Wheat Berries, and Rice
- Spirulina

COMPLEX CARBOHYDRATES

Carbohydrates often get a bad rap nowadays, just like fat did a few decades ago. However, the human diet requires balance in all aspects, and that includes carbohydrates. After all, this fuel source helps to supply the brain, nervous system, and red blood cells. Not only that, but grains, beans, and other sources of complex carbohydrates consume a large amount of protein, nutrients, and fiber.

If you want to stick to your vegan diet, then you need to focus on consuming a balance of all the delicious foods you can eat. This will both keep you fueled up on nutrients, but it will also prevent you from getting bored with your diet. The vegan lifestyle is meant to be fun, exciting, and delicious. You can only achieve this if you focus on incorporating a variety of flavors and textures into your daily meals.

OTHER NUTRIENTS

By consuming a balanced diet, you will naturally consume most, if not all, of the nutrients the human body requires. However, there are a few types of nutrients you should stay especially aware of on the vegan diet, as they are not as easy to come by in plant-based sources. Thankfully, there are plenty of resources to help vegans stay healthy today. For instance, you should consider taking a vegan multivitamin. There are plenty of these vitamins on the market, but you should always research the brand to ensure it is high quality. While there are many great options that you can buy both online and in-stores, one I personally prefer is Deva's Vegan Multivitamin.

Omega-3 fatty acids are a type of vital fat that decreases inflammation and aging while improving overall health. Sadly, most people in western countries do not consume enough of this fat, largely because it is most densely found in fish. However, you can still get omega-3 fats on a vegan diet, such as in flaxseeds, walnuts, seaweed and algae, hemp, and soy products. You can also purchase omega-3 supplements produced with algae, which has been found to be more effective and easier on the stomach than fish-derived supplements. One great brand is Freshfields's Vegan Omega-3.

Vitamin B-12 is not usually found in plant-based foods; however, you can get your daily supply through nutritional yeast and fortified ingredients such as grains, dairy-free milk, and soy products. Dairy-free milk, such as soy or almond milk, are often fortified; however, you should read the label to ensure your preferred brand is one of the fortified options. Of course, you can also get added B-12 in your daily vitamin.

Surprising to many people is that you don't need dairy to consume calcium. Not only that, but just as important for your bone health as calcium is vitamin D, as you cannot absorb and utilize the calcium unless you also have adequate vitamin D levels. Sadly, while many people consume more than enough calcium, many individuals in Western countries are deficient in vitamin D. While you can get this important vitamin in your daily vitamins, you can also get your daily requirements simply by spending thirty minutes out in the sunlight every day.

Macronutrients or macros and micronutrients or micros are molecules that the human body needs to survive, properly function and avoid getting ill. We need macros in large amounts as they are the primary nutrients for our body. There are three main macronutrients: carbohydrates, proteins, and fats.

WATER

Water makes up a considerable part of our bodies. It manages our body temperature level and helps in the metabolic process.

The Institute of Medicine suggests drinking 13 cups of water (more or less 3 liters) for males and 9 cups (or 2.2 liters) for females. Not sure if you are getting enough water?

Should you count macronutrients instead of calories?

Thinking that calories are the typical means to evaluate your food consumption, why would you take into consideration switching over to grams of macronutrients? The main factor that calories aren't excellent for determining just how healthy and balanced your food options are is that they do not take into consideration what you are consuming. 100 calories of broccoli will certainly rate the exact same as 100 calories of cake, though the 2 could not be more different from a nutritional standpoint.

Changing over to counting your macros, on the other hand, takes top quality food and satiation right into account. By tracking your macro needs, you have a much better possibility of complying with a diet plan that makes good sense for your health and wellness.

Just how to figure out your macronutrient requirements

While nutritional experts advise particular proportions of each macronutrient for ideal health and wellness, every person's dietary demands will certainly be various. You can identify your specific macronutrient levels with these actions.

1. Identify your calorie requirements:

Your day-to-day calorie requirements depend on lots of variables, including your age, weight, physical fitness level, and a lot more. You can establish your degrees by tracking what you consume in an ordinary week (one in which you aren't shedding or getting weight). The ordinary degree from nowadays is an excellent indication of your calorie requirements.

2. Transform calorie counts to macronutrients

You can designate these calories in the direction of macronutrients based on the proportion you are following when you understand your calorie targets. Frequently, the macronutrient intakes varies between (AMDR) 45-

65% of your day-to-day calories from carbohydrates, 20-35% from fats, and 10-35% from healthy protein.

Next off, you can identify the variety of grams to you readily available with standard mathematics. Right here's an instance:

By thinking you require 2,000 calories daily, you can establish your fat consumption by increasing 2,000 by 0.20 (the proportion of fat for 40:40:20 macronutrient divides). That completes 400, which is the variety of daily calories to dedicate to nutritional fat. To establish your gram consumption, divide 400 by 9 (the calories in a gram of fat) for a complete need of 44 grams of fat daily.

Chapter 7.
How to Get the Right Amount of Protein and Other Benefits from A Vegetarian Diet?

First, let's explain that the concept of nutrition for a vegan bodybuilder involves not only adequate protein intake, calorie control, and fat dosage. This is a certain system in which success depends literally on everything: the frequency of food intake, the total amount of proteins and dietary supplements are taken, the amount of fluid consumed, the combination of products and many other factors.

From how rationally the bodybuilder himself will be able to organize his diet - from the number of meals to the amount of water drunk - its result directly depends on a number of factors. Success, in this case, is a derivative of an integrated approach, and not just the influence of protein, as the followers of meat-eating believe.

CHOOSE YOUR TYPE OF NUTRITION

You must understand the difference between vegetarianism and veganism. Only you can decide what type of nutrition (lacto-, ovo-, lasto+ovo-, vegetarianism or strict veganism) is most suitable for you personally and corresponds to your lifestyle.

EAT REAL FOOD

Forget about processed artificial food and gradually switch to natural: only from such food can the body draw strength and energy for itself.

Whole foods like nuts, legumes, vegetables, and seeds have enough nutrients that the muscles require and provide a steady supply of blood glucose and amino acid to muscles, unlike the nutritional dreck sold at the local supermarket.

Refuse fried foods in favor of cooked ones - this will greatly help your body and muscles.

TRACK YOUR INTAKE

The only possible way to find out if you are consuming foods adequately in the balanced proportions to develop the muscle is to record a fully detailed food diary and tally your macronutrients and calories.

Consult your trainer or nutritionist before making changes to your diet and trying to gain weight.

Calculate your daily calorie intake. When losing weight, people create a calorie deficit, that is, they burn more calories with their activity than they eat with food. To gain weight, you need to do the opposite: you need to get more calories with food than will be spent during the day. Ask your trainer for the correct calorie calculation just for you.

Consult your trainer or nutritionist before making changes to your diet and trying to gain weight.

EAT ENOUGH CALORIES

The muscle is known to be a metabolically active tissue; therefore, you have to consume plenty of calories to keep it growing. If you aim to gain weight, consume around 20 calories for each pound of body weight daily. If you discover that 20 calories for each pound gathers fat and mass, come down to 15–17 calories. But this doesn't imply that you can consume pound pizzas. Quality is essential, therefore keep it clean.

DON'T SHUN CARBS

Half of the calories consumed per day should be carbohydrates - this is the "fuel" for the muscles.

To gain weight, you have to consume a lot of carbohydrates: about 3g for each pound of body weight. They contain glycogen to help with the intense lifting and calories needed for growth. Meals like brown rice, quinoa, oatmeal, and sweet potatoes are great options.

DON'T SHUN FATS

Fats are needed to deliver energy to muscles during training. The traditional bodybuilding diet for gaining muscle mass suggests that 20% of the total calorie intake should be composed of fat. Good sources of fats are olive oil, almonds, walnuts, avocados.

PACK IN PROTEIN

Protein gives the amino acids which are used in developing the muscle. Opt for 1–1.6g of protein for each pound of body weight, or 180–270g a daily for a 180-pounder. We told you about the best plant protein options above. These products provide muscles with adequate amino acids for growth and recovery.

Mix various foods that contain protein: beans, nuts, lentils, chickpeas, peas, *seitan* (vegetable meat), greens, seeds, sesame seeds, soy milk, tofu, quinoa. Then your body will receive the full range of amino acids necessary for muscle growth.

RISE & DINE

When aiming to gain mass, consume 2 breakfasts. This will help you refill your liver glycogen and put a stop to the catabolism which chips away overnight, take in 2 scoops of whey protein, and a fast-digesting carb-like fresh fruit or smoothie after waking. After about 60 minutes, consume wholefoods breakfast that contains adequate protein—like beans, pulses, lentils, chickpeas, tofu, edamame, tempeh —and slower-burning carbs, like oatmeal.

DO NOT SKIP MEALS

Eat 5-6 times a day, in small portions. Your daily meal should consist of breakfast, lunch, dinner and two or three healthy snacks.

Make sure at least one portion of green salad per day is present in your diet - the amino acids contained in it will contribute to muscle growth.

Also, eat fruit for breakfast - this will not only give your body useful substances but also wake it up, stimulating it to act. After all, for an athlete starting the day right is the key to a successful day!

DRINK PLENTY OF WATER REGULARLY

You need to drink a lot of water - at least 8-10 glasses a day. You can also get a good amount of calories with fluid. Use soft tofu, soaked nuts, seeds, and unrefined oils. Just add them to your smoothie!

MUNCH BEFORE BED

Before going to bed, consume some healthy fat and protein smoothie. As you sleep, proteins will slow catabolism by supplying a steady amount of amino acids About 40 minutes before you sleep, eat a cup of tempeh or tofu combined with 2tbsp of flaxseed oil or 2 ounces of seeds or nuts.

MODE OF TRAINING AND REST

To gain muscle mass, you need a good sleep and rest, because the muscles grow at this time, and not during training.

ADD NUTRITIONAL SUPPLEMENTS IF NECESSARY

If you notice cramping in your legs during exercise or at night, then you are short of sodium and potassium. Try to increase the intake of these elements in the body - for example, nutritional supplements will help.

If you are troubled by sleep problems, add zinc and magnesium to your diet, which will help your body relax after exhausting workouts.

Pay special attention to foods that are rich in iron, zinc, calcium, vitamins D and B12, as well as omega-3 acids.

PLAN AHEAD

Getting back from a workout session, tired and exhausted can tempt you to consume foods you shouldn't. But preparing enough protein-packed meals which can easily be microwaved will lead you to make healthy choices and gain the nutrients needed by your muscles. Make good use of your weekends to prepare big batches of hard-boiled eggs, chicken (if you are an ovo-vegetarian or have not entirely excluded animal products from your diet), rice, chili and stews, which can be frozen for the whole week.

Chapter 8.
The Best Proteins That a Bodybuilder Should Know

Think it or not, you can really prosper, and never ever endure a healthy protein shortage on a plant-based diet. Since you should consider precisely how energetic your way of living is, a well-thought whole food plant-based diet regimen offers even more than sufficient healthy protein to please the body's demands without all the artery-clogging saturated fats that are present in the current American diet plan.

As a vegan endurance professional athlete, I put a high-stress level on my body. I have to admit my plant-based diet plan has sustained me for years without any adverse effect on structure, lean muscular tissue mass, or recuperation.

Healthy protein is composed of parts called amino acids. Throughout food digestion, your body will certainly break down the healthy protein right into these amino acids and will utilize them for various processes in your body. A few of these uses consist of constructing bones, muscle mass, and various other body cells, producing hormonal agents, and sustaining natural chemical features.

There are 22 amino acids, 9 of which your body cannot make, so they should be acquired from your diet plan. These are generally called vital amino acids.

Numerous plant-based healthy protein resources have some, yet not every one of the crucial amino acids. This makes it essential to consume a range of these vegetarian or vegan foods throughout the day.

LIST OF TOP PLANT-BASED FOODS HIGH IN PROTEIN

Quinoa

A grain-like seed, quinoa is a great healthy protein choice that can be substituted to rice or pasta, offered alone or over greens and vegetables. It can be 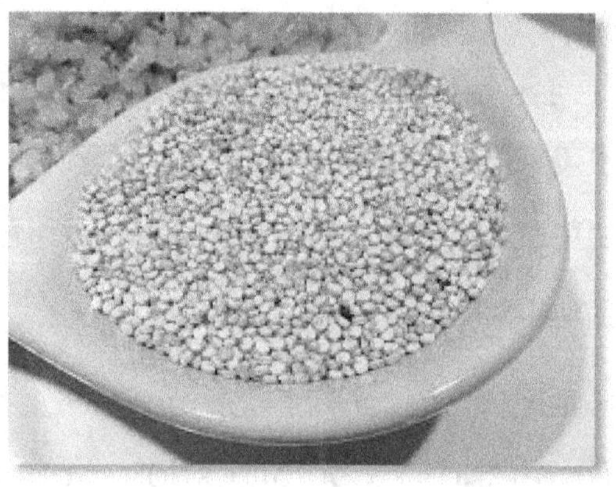 offered cool with almond or with coconut milk and berries, it provides an excellent base for a veggie burger and is likewise an amazing morning meal grain.

Lentils

These beans provide intricate carbs for continual power and well-balanced blood glucose levels. The soluble fiber they have feed excellent germs in the gut fundamental for us because they aid at maintain us healthy and balanced and might reduce cholesterol, overall and LDL (frequently called "negative" cholesterol). Lentils are abundant in iron, as well.

At 18 grams of healthy protein per prepared cup (240 ml), lentils are an excellent resource of healthy protein.

They can be used in a range of recipes, varying from fresh salads to spice-infused dahls and hearty soups.

Lentils additionally have excellent quantities of gradually absorbed carbohydrates, and a single cup (240 ml) supplies about 50% of your suggested everyday fiber consumption.

The kind of fiber found in lentils has been revealed to feed the great microorganisms in your colon, advertising a healthy and balanced digestive tract. Lentils might additionally help in reducing the danger of heart problems, diabetes mellitus, excess body weight, and some kinds of cancer cells.

Additionally, lentils are abundant in manganese, folate, and iron. They additionally include an excellent quantity of antioxidants and various other health-promoting plant substances.

Lentils are dietary giants. They are abundant in healthy protein and consist of great quantities of various other nutrients. They might likewise help in reducing the danger of numerous illnesses.

Walnuts

Unlike various other nuts, walnuts include a considerable quantity of the omega-3 fat referred to as alpha-linolenic acid (ALA), 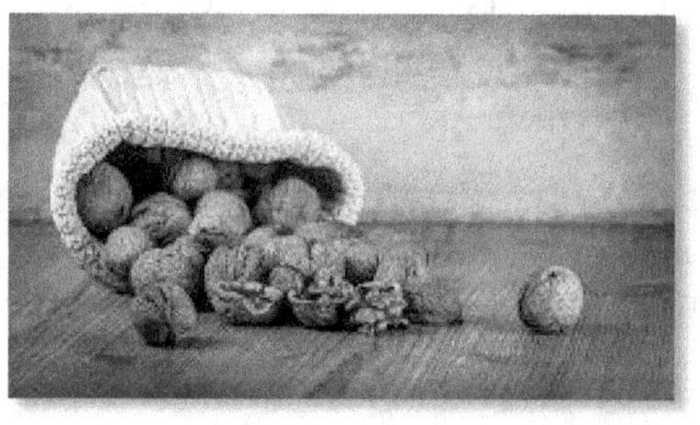 which aids the heart and the mind. They likewise flaunt extra antioxidant power than various other nuts, assisting to shield the body from totally free extreme damages. Walnuts have been revealed to enhance cognitive features.

Maca powder

This superfood invigorates without being an energizer and contains significant amounts of vitamin C, calcium, potassium, and magnesium. Maca aids to preserve the balance, and the equilibrium of the body lowers anxiety levels, and it might relieve anxiety and anxiousness.

Chia seeds

Chia seeds are stemmed from the Salvia hispanica plant, which grows both in Mexico and Guatemala.

At 6 grams of healthy protein and 13 grams of fiber per 1.25 ounces (35 grams), chia seeds certainly deserve their spot on this checklist.

What's even more, these little seeds consist of a great quantity of iron, magnesium, calcium, and selenium, along with omega-3 fats, antioxidants, and numerous other advantageous plant substances.

They're likewise extremely flexible. Chia seeds have this peculiar quality of becoming a gel-like compound if immersed and let to get soaked in water or any other liquid. This makes them a very easy enhancement to a selection of dishes, varying from smoothie mixes to baked products and chia desserts.

Chia seeds are a useful resource of plant healthy protein. They additionally consist of a range of vitamins, minerals, antioxidants, and various other health-promoting substances.

Flaxseeds

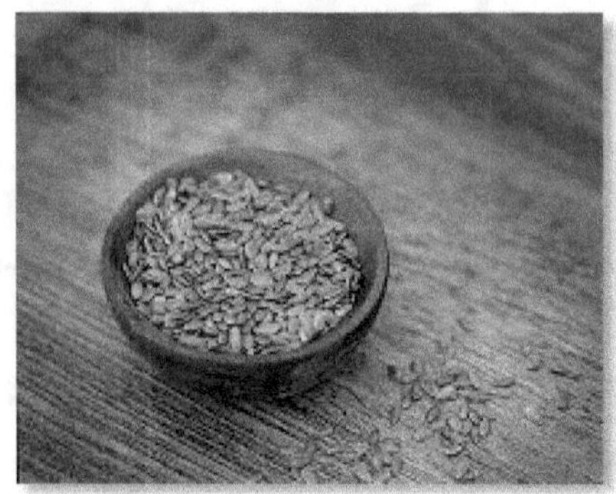

These seeds have the highest degree of omega-3 fat alpha-linolenic acid (ALA) of all plant foods, along with an optimal proportion of omega-3 to omega-6 fats. Flaxseeds aid the equilibrium of estrogen levels, ease menopausal signs and have resulted to boost the prostate-cancer defense. In individuals with coronary artery conditions, they have been located to enhance triglyceride levels and high blood pressure.

Hempseed

Hempseed originates from the Cannabis sativa plant, which is infamous for coming from the very same family as the cannabis plant.

Hempseed has just trace quantities of THC, the substance that creates the marijuana-like medication results.

Not as widely known as various other seeds, hempseed contains 10 grams of the total, conveniently absorbable healthy protein per ounce (28 grams). That's 50% greater than chia seeds and flaxseeds.

Hempseed likewise has an excellent quantity of magnesium, iron, zinc, calcium, and selenium. What's even more, it is an excellent resource of omega-3 and omega-6 fats in the proportion thought to be optimum for human health and wellness.

Surprisingly, some researches show that the sort of fats located in hempseed might help in reducing swelling, along with reducing signs of PMS, menopause, and particular skin diseases.

You can include hemp seed to your diet regimen by scattering some in your smoothie mix or early morning muesli. It can likewise be utilized in homemade salad dressings or healthy protein bars.

Hempseed consists of an excellent quantity of total, highly digestible healthy protein, in addition to health-promoting vital fats in a proportion optimum for human health and wellness.

Spirulina

This turquoise alga is absolutely a dietary giant.

2 tablespoons (30 ml) give you 8 grams of total healthy protein, along with covering 22% of your everyday demands of iron and thiamin, and 42% of your daily copper requirements.

Spirulina, moreover, has good quantities of magnesium, riboflavin, manganese, potassium, and high percentages of a lot of the various other nutrients your body demands, consisting of crucial fats.

Phycocyanin, an all-natural pigment located in spirulina, shows up to have effective antioxidant, anti-cancer, and anti-inflammatory residential properties Researches connect taking in spirulina to wellness advantages varying from a more robust immune system, minimized blood stress to improve blood sugar and cholesterol levels.

Spirulina is a nutritious, high-protein food with lots of advantageous health-enhancing buildings.

Ezekiel bread and various other kinds of bread made from sprouted grains

Ezekiel bread is made from natural, grew whole grains and beans. These breads are made of wheat, millet, barley, and spelt, along with lentils and soybeans.

2 pieces of Ezekiel bread have about 8 grams of healthy protein, which is somewhat greater than the ordinary Bread.

Growing vegetables, and grains, enhances the quantity of healthy and balanced nutrients they consist of and decreases the number of anti-nutrients in them.

On top of that, research studies reveal that rising increases their amino acid material. Lysine is the limiting amino acid in several plants and rising boosts the lysine net content - this aids in improving the total healthy protein of high quality.

Soymilk

Milk that's made from soybeans and strengthened with minerals, and vitamins, is a wonderful alternative to cow's milk.

It does not it include just 7 grams of healthy protein per cup (240 ml), yet, it is likewise an outstanding resource of calcium, vitamin D and vitamin B12

Keep in mind that soymilk and soybeans do not normally consist of vitamin B12, so choosing a strengthened range is advised.

Soymilk is found in a lot of grocery stores. It is an exceptionally functional product that can be eaten by itself or added to a range of food preparation and cooking recipes.

It is a great suggestion to select bitter ranges to maintain the quantity of sugar to a minimum.

Soymilk is a high-protein plant option to cow's milk. It is a flexible item that can be made use of in a selection of means.

Oats and oatmeal

Oats are a tasty and very easy food to include in a diet plan, and it is an excellent source of plant-based healthy protein.

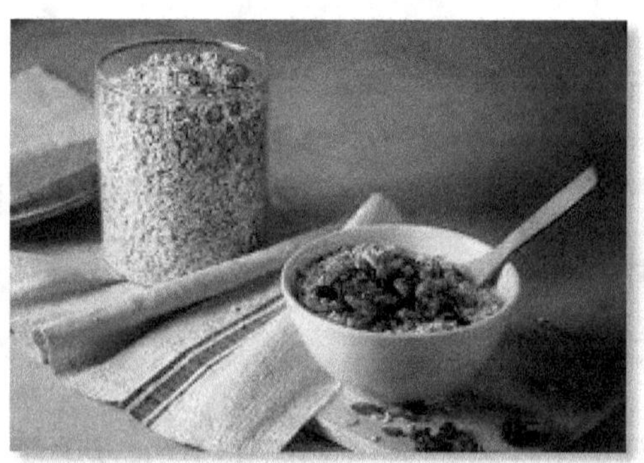

Fifty percent of a cup (120 ml) of completely dry oats gives you about 6 grams of healthy protein and 4 grams of fiber. This portion additionally includes great quantities of magnesium, zinc, folate, and phosphorus.

Oats are not taken into consideration a full, healthy protein, but it does include higher-quality healthy protein than various other frequently eaten grains like rice and wheat.

You can make use of oats in a selection of dishes varying from oatmeal to veggie hamburgers. They can be grounded directly into the flour and used for cooking.

Oats are not just nourishing yet additionally a tasty and a very easy method to include plant healthy protein right into a vegan or vegetarian diet regimen.

Basmati rice

Basmati rice consists of about 1.5 times as much healthy protein as various other long-grain rice selections, consisting of wild rice and basmati.

One prepared cup (240 ml) gives 7 grams of healthy protein, along with a great quantity of fiber, manganese, magnesium, phosphorus, vitamin b, and copper.

Unlike white rice, basmati rice is not removed from its bran. This is excellent from a dietary viewpoint, as bran includes fiber and a lot of minerals and vitamins.

This creates issues concerning arsenic, which can build up in the bran of rice plants expanded in contaminated locations. Arsenic is a poisonous micronutrient that might trigger different illnesses, particularly when consumed consistently for extended periods of time. Cleaning basmati rice before the food preparation and its use is fundamental, so use a lot of water to steam it - this might minimize the arsenic content by as much as 57%.

Basmati rice is a yummy, nutrient-rich plant resource of healthy protein. Those depending on basmati rice as a food staple must take safety measures to decrease its arsenic net content.

Chapter 9.
Vegetarian Bodybuilding Diet Plan

BREAKFAST:

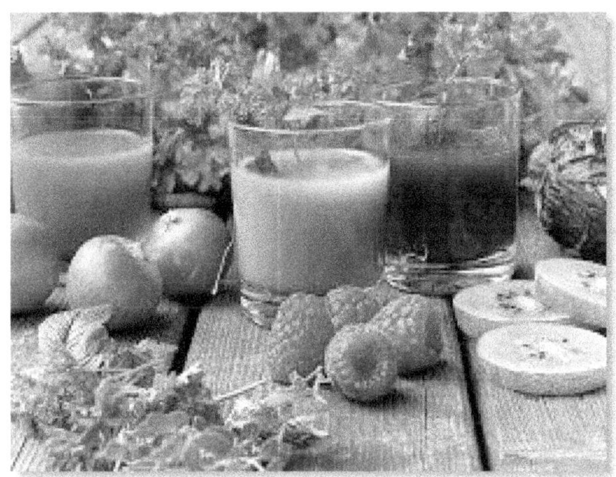

- Freshly squeezed vegetable or fruit juice
- At least three slices of whole-grain bread
- Peanut butter
- Muddle can be cooked with cow's milk or its substitutes

A SNACK:

- Vegetable casserole
- Nuts, preferably a mixture

LUNCH:

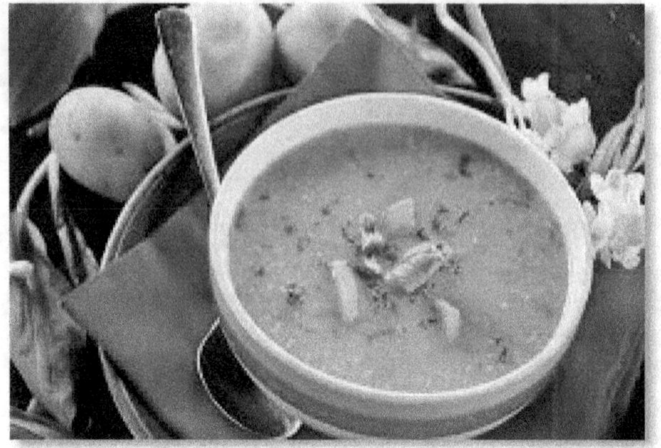

- Vegetable soup
- Stewed vegetables
- Soybean meal
- Pace

A SNACK:

- Skimmed kefir (Cultured Butter milk)
- Seeds
- Jem's a fruit
- A piece of bread

DINNER:

- Boiled potatoes, mashed potatoes
- Cheese

- Broccoli boiled or steamed
- Half an avocado
- Tofu

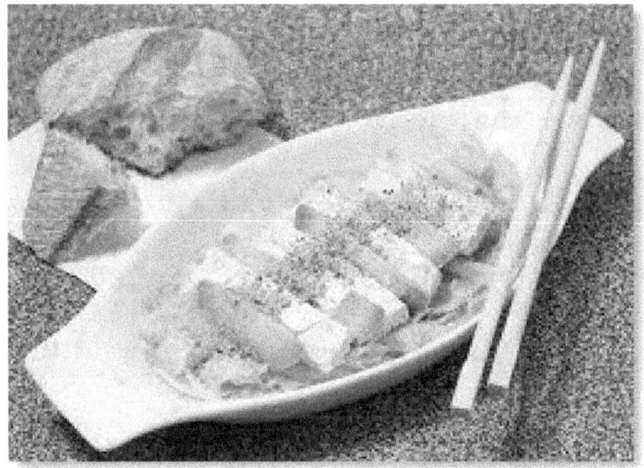

VEGETARIAN'S DINING TABLE

Vegetarian bodybuilders need to include vegetarians in their diet and sports supplements, but they should not be the leading protein supplier. One half of the daily dose of protein derived from the supplements and the other half should be derived from the food.

How vegetarianism will affect your health:

Lowering your sugar level

Strengthening immunity

Complete removal of slag and toxins

Vessel improvement

Cholesterol reduction

Doctors have different views on the harm and benefits of vegetarianism.

Vegetarian diets may be prescribed for the treatment or prevention of certain diseases.

Before switching to a plant-based diet, a nutritionist should be consulted.

Take the necessary tests, undergo a full examination.

Together with a specialist will determine the necessary set of products

Create a detailed menu.

Develop a smooth transition to a vegetable type of food.

Milk, eggs, and honey will be a mandatory recommendation from all physicians.

Chapter 10.
Foods to Avoid in Our Diet and Unhealthy Eating Habits

Becoming a vegan seems simple enough. It would seem enough to avoid animal products - what could be easier? But this is not so. Many foods purchased in the store contain ingredients that either contain substances of animal origin, or, in one way or another, are associated with the exploitation of animals. In short, there are many foods that seem vegan, but vegans should avoid them.

Besides the commonly understood vegan no-nos, foods to say goodbye to forever include:

- All meat, poultry, and animal flesh;
- Seafood;
- Dairy products;
- Bee produced products like honey, beeswax, royal jelly, and pollen;
- Food additives: some of them of animal origin;
- Dairy ingredients: whey, casein, and lactose are obtained only from dairy products;
- Chips (may contain chicken fat or dairy ingredients such as casein, whey or animal-derived enzymes);

- White sugar, brown sugar, powdered sugar (it is better to replace them with maple syrup or agave nectar as a sweetener);
- Some varieties of dark chocolate (contain animal products - whey, milk fat, milk powder, refined oil or skimmed milk powder);
- Red products that owe their color to red pigments obtained from the bodies of cochineal females (insects). On the label, this ingredient is labeled cochineal, carmine acid, or carmine;
- Margarine (may contain gelatin, casein (milk protein) and whey);
- Pasta (some types of pasta, especially fresh ones, contain eggs);
- Non-dairy cream (many varieties of such cream contain milk protein casein);
- Worcestershire sauce (spicy soy sauce with vinegar and spices): many varieties contain anchovies;
- Gelatin (a product of the processing of connective tissue of animals);
- Pepsin (the enzyme is present in the gastric juice of mammals, birds, reptiles and most fish);
- Vitamin d3 (most vitamin d3 is derived from fish oil or lanolin, which is present in sheep's wool);

- Omega-3 fatty acids (the source of most omega-3s is fish).

Even seemingly safe 'vitamins' can have animal origins or derivatives. As a vegan, you will get used to reading labels. In many countries, it is a legal requirement to declare specific ingredients, and this is definitely the case when animal products are involved.

Chapter 11.
Supplements for The Vegetarian Bodybuilder

There are times when the body has increased needs, due to an intense training or competition schedule. It is for these times that supplements are an invaluable asset to athletes who want their performance to be at an all-time high. Thankfully, there are many supplements that are appropriate for the vegan diet.

But how do supplements actually work? What happens when you swallow that pill? Simply put, the active ingredients contained within the supplement are released into the stomach after you swallow them. From here they pass through the small intestine before being distributed throughout the bloodstream. When the body breaks down the nutrients it is, when the majority of supplements fail. Stomach acids easily destroy poor-quality nutrient supplements, leaving you with an absorption rate of less than 10%. Choosing high-quality supplements is beyond essential!

THE 4 MOST IMPORTANT FACTORS TO CONSIDER WHEN CHOOSING HEALTH SUPPLEMENTS

To make sure that you are getting the optimum results from your health supplements, pay attention to these 4 factors when you go shopping!

Bioavailability: The higher the absorption rate of the supplement, the better it is. They are of no use to the body if no absorption occurs. Liquid nutritional supplements offer the best absorption rate.

All-Natural: Look at the ingredient list carefully. Search for supplements which have no added artificial preservatives, allergens, or dyes. Keeping your supplements as all-natural as possible is the ultimate goal.

Tested in the Lab: Reputable companies will stand behind their products and submit to testing done not only by their in-house labs, but also by independents.

Calcium

Calcium is essential for the formation of stronger bones that athletes in particular need. High-performance athletes put a huge amount of stress on their bones so, in order to ensure that breaks do not occur, calcium supplements are available in various strengths.

Iron

Iron can be a difficult mineral to get enough of. It is a part of every cell in the body and is responsible for carrying oxygen from the lungs to other parts of the body. This is a vital mineral for athletes.

Zinc

Athletes require zinc for numerous functions throughout the body, but mostly for proper workings of bones and muscles. The bioavailability of zinc, when obtained from plant sources is said to be less than from meat and dairy. To ensure that your body does not run out of this trace mineral, it is recommended for athletes that a supplement is taken.

Protein Powders

While plenty of protein can be found in the vegan diet, these powders are a good way to get some extra protein when it is needed quickly. For example, in the morning or right after training. They mix easily with water or juice and are available in a number of flavors.

"B" Vitamins

There are 8 different groups of B-Vitamins, and they are more than essential for athletes since they are needed for energy production and red blood cell production. They are also known as the "stress" vitamin.

Vitamin C

While this may seem to be surprising, not all vegans are major fruit lovers. While fruit is known as the best source of Vitamin C, it is also prevalent in vegetables. Even though more than enough can be found in vegetables, in order to ensure that you are keeping up a steady supply in your body a supplement may be a good idea. There are several forms of Vitamin C available. Any extra Vitamin C that has been consumed, but not used by the body, will be excreted in the urine.

Evidence has shown that many high performing professional and amateur athletes experience lower immune competence (weakened immune systems). This is usually accompanied by frequent infection of the upper respiratory tract.

Such symptoms are usually the result of prolonged stress from regular high-intensity training. Similarly, a short period of intense exercise creates a temporary reduction in immune function. Some of the properties of the immune system reduced by high-intensity training include neutrophil function and the natural cell degeneration number.

Intense workouts have a negative effect on the neutrophil function (white blood cells) and this can lead to poor immune-response and increase in microbial infections. Consequently, it will lead to a disruption in training and affect the athlete's performance. Coaches and trainers, who work with top professional and amateur athletes, usually want training to be continuous without any interruptions due to illness caused by viral infections. That is why it is beneficial for all dedicated athletes who adopt a vegan diet to choose foods that will effectively boost immune competence. Thus, the athlete will be able to enjoy continuous training without disruptions due to illness.

EFFECT OF FATTY FOODS ON IMMUNE-COMPETENCE

Poorly planned diets and consumption of a high amount of fatty food can worsen the immune suppression caused by intense exercise. But when athletes take a sufficient quantity of micronutrients such as selenium, iron, copper, zinc, Vitamin B6, B12, C, and E, carotenoids, and folate, the effect of the immune suppression will be drastically reduced. The body's immune function is greatly enhanced by carotenoids, which are pigment molecules available in large quantity in green and colored vegetables.

Unfortunately, the typical modern diet has an excess of omega-6 fatty acid – a type of polyunsaturated fatty acid that causes chronic inflammation. Research has shown that omega-3 fatty acid, which is commonly found in seeds of sunflower, pumpkin, sesame, hemp and flax plants, is healthier than fats and oils derived from animal sources. These seeds also provide amino acids (the building blocks of protein) and healthy fat. The appropriate amount of fatty acids, sterols, lignans and other nutrients improves the immune competence of the body.

PLANT BASED ANTIOXIDANTS VS ANTIOXIDANT SUPPLEMENTS

A diet with relatively high quantity of phytochemicals (chemical compounds that occur naturally in plants) and antioxidants can also reduce oxidative stress caused by intense training. Just one bout of an intense workout can produce a significant amount of oxidative stress in the muscles and blood stream. This may stay on for a couple of days during which the endogenous antioxidant defenses are increased. On the contrary, reactive oxygen species (ROS) created by the intense workout may outweigh the increase in endogenous antioxidants. But regular consumption of high-antioxidant plant-based foods keeps ROS at desirable levels and reduces the negative effects of oxidative stress.

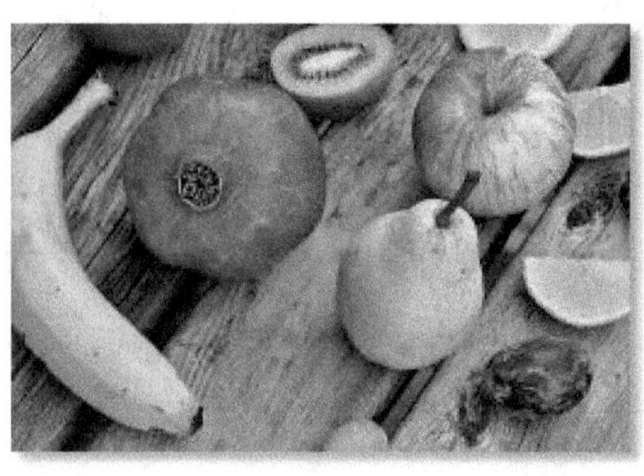

But it is important to note that antioxidant supplements have not produced predictable results when used to reduce oxidative stress induced by intense training or to curtail inflammatory markers. In some cases, these supplements have actually slowed down recovery. In one study, creatine kinase, which is a major indicator of muscle damage, remained at a high level for a longer period than those who were given a placebo.

In a second study, administering a concentrated antioxidant to the participants raised lipid peroxidation and reduced the level of glutathione peroxidase – an antioxidant enzyme. Other reports and some studies of chronic diseases show that high micronutrient whole foods, which contain complex mixtures of phyto-nutrients and antioxidants, are more potent than supplements containing high doses of isolated antioxidants. There is also strong evidence showing that vegetables protect the body against coronary heart failure which also involves oxidative damage. But the benefit of using antioxidant vitamin supplements to prevent this disease is not clear.

Broccoli, collards, kale, bok choy and other green vegetables, provide a significantly higher quantity of micronutrients per kilocalorie than other foods. They also contain protein. Virtually all colorful vegetables are rich in antioxidants. In addition, fruits like kiwi, oranges, sour cherries, pomegranates, berries and black currants, have high quantities of antioxidants. Seeds like black unhulled sesame seed and pistachio nuts also have high amounts of antioxidants including vitamin E.

Chapter 12.
Vegan's Guide for Athletic Training

The hardest part of getting started is just knowing where to start! Many people know they want to be fit. This is one of the most common new year's resolutions, but meeting that need is an entirely different problem.

If you're worried about joining a gym, start buying some home weight. It's okay to start with small steps. When it comes to bodybuilding, rest a lot better. Soon enough, it can cause you injuries that can make you thoroughly discouraged. The more disciplined you are, the faster you can change your exercise routine to meet your personal needs.

Growth rates depend on several factors: genetics, speed of recovery, metabolic rate, environmental factors, food and water, sleep or injury. So don't be disappointed if your growth rate is slower than you initially thought.

Bodybuilding brings you to many beautiful things in your life. Not only does it help you look better and feel more secure, it also has fantastic health benefits.

- Reduces the risk of premature death (even from heart disease).

- Reduces the risk of diabetes.
- Reduces the risk of high blood pressure (or high blood pressure if you already have one).
- Reduces the risk of colon cancer.
- Reduces the feeling of depression and anxiety.
- It helps control your weight.
- Helps build and maintain healthy bones, muscles and joints.
- Promotes psychological well-being.
- It promotes a better dream.
- Promotes a better sex life.
- Help improve your memory.

Despite all the health benefits and all the benefits of a vegan diet, there is no end to achieving that goal.

If you've been involved with bodybuilding (or fitness in general) before, you've already overcome the first major hurdles. This guide can guide you in the right direction to ensure that your diet and exercise plan is proper for you!

Creating a Successful Training Program

Choosing the right exercise program for you can be a daunting task. There are many available, so before adding yourself to endless information, consider the following:

Your skill level: To avoid injury, you need to think seriously about your body's ability. If you are new to exercise or come back after a long time, you want to introduce yourself slowly.

Consider this beginner's routine for your first day:

Workout:

- Warm-Up Stretches
- Squats – 10 Reps
- Bench Presses – 10 Reps
- Chin Pulldowns – 10 Reps
- Standing Calf Raises – 10 Reps
- Back Extensions – 10 Reps
- Crunches – 10 Reps
- Lunges – 10 Reps
- Cool Down Cardio – 20 minutes walking.

Cardiovascular, stretching and warm-up exercises are very important, you can't stress enough. If you do not complete this part of your training, you are at risk of injury and your recovery time will be much longer. Walking is preferable to running because running can be a waste of time in the wrong places.

Your Resistance: This will improve your workouts as much as you can, but as a starting point you should consider the last time you did this activity: Did it affect you for the next few days or the next day well? Was? This should indicate how much your body can handle the exercise. The bodybuilding exercises are short but intense, and if you do not give yourself enough time to rest, you will be injured.

Your goal: Is your goal to gain weight, lose weight or gain strength? There are programs designed for a wide variety of purposes, so once you decide what you want to do, it will be easy to find a nutrition and training program.

Your availability: You need to have a realistic view of the amount of time you have to spend at the gym. If you choose a program that you do more than you can do, you are doomed from the start. It is best to start with a 3 to the 4-day program to get motivated but does not worry about your new lifestyle.

Equipment: You should see what the gym offers, or if you can't go to the gym regularly, you don't have what you can have at home. Including equipment in your plan that you do not have access to means a disaster.

Your preferences: you want to enjoy exercising, so consider the exercises that appeal to you to make sure your bodybuilding program is implemented.

Muscle Fibers

Rapid torsion muscle fibers have always been associated with runners and lifters, but they can also be beneficial for bodybuilding. The human body is equipped with a full range of muscle fibers. From smaller rotating fibers with resistance and slow elastic fibers to faster and larger. Rapid torsion fibers store a lot of carbohydrates and water, so maximizing them, you will find a more complete and dense appearance.

A lot of balance between fast and slow contraction muscle fibers is reduced to your genes, but you can still organize your training regimen to maximize strength and growth. There are two ways to do this: the amount of weight you lift and how you manage your fatigue.

The higher the weight you lift and the more pressure you exert on your body, the higher the rotation fibers, so you may want to add more weight to the lower series of repetitions to gain more weight. Consider a training schedule

You will also want to tire your slow stretch fibers so that your body works the tissues of your spin instead. The way to achieve this is to keep the intensity of your training high. Instead of taking an hour to do 15 sets of specific training, shorten your breaks and do not pause if the movement is difficult and do not maintain your 15-hour training for half an hour. In doing so, the twisted fibers will force you to kick.

Some excellent exercises to do this are the exercises that want the most muscle:

Squat, dead-end, breast press, shoulder press, immersion, stretching, etc.

Do this in smaller but more intense series and try to stop the movements without taking pain into account.

HOME EXERCISES ESSENTIAL FOR YOUR SUCCESS

There are many bodybuilding exercises you can do at home, without the necessary equipment! If you can't always go to the gym but still want to continue, these are essential, but there are things you can do.

Here is an example of Work Home Out:

The chest

- Medium press additives: 3 sets, 6 to 8 repetitions.
- Extensive increase in pressure: 3 sets, 6 to 8 repetitions.

- Medium pressure (long legs): 3 sets, 6 to 8 repetitions.
- Broad Grip Press Ups (long legs): 3 sets, 6 to 8 repetitions.

Triceps

This is included in your chest training, but if you want to do more, you can always include foreground presses.

Back

- Upper back - pull up

Hyperextensions (with someone lowering their legs): 8 to 10 repetitions.

Biceps

In addition to stretching, you can find something at home that lifts weights.

The legs

Training your feet without equipment is difficult, but squatting, especially if you have something heavy, will be a way to help you.

Abs

- Sets of lies: 3 sets, 6 to 8 repetitions.
- Torsion screws: 3 sets, 6 to 8 repetitions.

- Normal kicks: 3 sets, 6 to 8 repetitions.

Shoulders

Your shoulders work when you make your press releases.

Aerobic exercises

Doing cardio out of exercise is easy. Running can be very difficult, although it affects your energy level and recovery time, so it is preferable to walk.

Conclusion

There are some essential things to keep in mind before starting vegan for athletic training, and you should keep them in mind throughout your training life:

Gradually, lift heavy weights: if you want to grow, you should continuously increase your activity or stay as simple as possible.

Protein should be consumed at 1 gram per pound of body weight; Protein is essential for athletes, especially if you follow a vegan diet. Always use protein powders if necessary.

- Sleep well: sleep helps with protein synthesis and muscle repair, so you should practice well enough during training.
- Positivity is the key: do not use it for mistakes and negative things that happen. Staying positive will keep you motivated and make your training more successful.
- Stress control: Cortisol is the body's most important stress hormone and uses proteins, so learning to manage stress is very important. Avoiding this is impossible, but you can be careful

and reduce (or quit smoking) and smoke, overcome negative thinking, containment and sleepless nights.

- Participate in aerobic exercises: walking lightly or doing cardio exercises helps your overall fitness and helps you stay fit until you work hard.

- Eat fats: Eating "good fats" is essential for your overall health, so you should include them in your diet.

- Avoid avoiding it: spending too much time will not give your body a chance to recover, which can cause injury. This can lead to a lack of motivation and health problems. Good ways to see overwhelming, fatigue, insomnia, thirst, loss of appetite, irritability, and decentralization.

- Supplements: to make sure you get everything you need; the supplements your diet lacks are perfect.

- Training: Keep up to date with the latest research and information on bodybuilding. New experiments are always performed and can still be applied to you.

Your vulnerability to protein deficiency depends mainly on your vegetarian diet. A careful vegetarian will not eat any animal protein source. They avoid not only animal meat but also fish, eggs, milk and eggs. A vegetarian generally avoids animal meat but may consume milk, eggs or fish. If you consume some animal protein, you probably consume enough animal protein. If you are a vegetarian, you are vulnerable to protein deficiency.

Many people prefer animal protein sources because of their digestibility. The body generally understands that plant protein sources are difficult to digest. They also contain less energy and less protein than animal products. Vegetarian athletes need to increase their overall protein intake to respond to this.

Another problem for vegetarian athletes is the amount of iron. Red meat is a much more significant source of iron than any vegetable protein source. Iron deficiency will cause numbness and reduced function. If you want to increase your iron intake while avoiding animal meat, drink coffee and tea with iron-rich foods, as this prevents absorption. Vitamin C, on the other hand, increases the body's ability to absorb iron. Occasionally, cook your fish in cast iron fish because there is evidence that it is washing your pan. Iron supplements are complicated because you don't want a lot of iron in your system.

For strict vegetarians, calcium intake can be a problem. Another thing to note: Calcium also absorbs iron. Take a look at the mix of sources from both. Also, if you are taking iron supplements as well as calcium supplements, you should be aware of your time. Take iron supplements with a meal or snack. But take calcium supplements only without food.

Hard vegetarians also face B12 deficiency, possibly because there is no plant source of this nutrient. If you're a strict vegan, you want to take a supplement or use a fortified soy product as your source.

The advantage of a vegan diet for athletes is that they tend to have a much more abundant protein, which is essential for the performance of the sport and the foundation of any exercise program.

Thanks, and enjoy it!

www.ingramcontent.com/pod-product-compliance
Lightning Source LLC
Chambersburg PA
CBHW070658250726

48662CB00001B/185